THE
HORMONE
BOOST

THE

HORMONE

BOOST

HOW TO
POWER UP YOUR
6 ESSENTIAL
HORMONES
FOR
STRENGTH,
ENERGY, AND
WEIGHT LOSS

DR. NATASHA TURNER
NATUROPATHIC DOCTOR

RODALE.

This book is intended as a reference volume only, not as a medical manual.
The information given here is designed to help you make informed decisions
about your health. It is not intended as a substitute for any treatment that
may have been prescribed by your doctor. If you suspect that you have a
medical problem, we urge you to seek competent medical help.

Mention of specific companies, organizations, or authorities in this book
does not imply endorsement by the author or publisher, nor does
mention of specific companies, organizations, or authorities imply
that they endorse this book, its author, or the publisher.

Internet addresses and telephone numbers given in this book
were accurate at the time it went to press.

This book is being published simultaneously in Canada by Random House Canada.

Rodale books may be purchased for business or promotional use
or for special sales. For information, please write to:
Special Markets Department, Rodale, Inc., 733 Third Avenue, New York, NY 10017

Printed in the United States of America
Rodale Inc. makes every effort to use acid-free ∞, recycled paper ♲.

Book design by Rachel Cooper

Library of Congress Cataloging-in-Publication Data is on file with the publisher.

ISBN-13 978-1-62336-677-3 hardcover

Distributed to the trade by Macmillan

2   4   6   8   10   9   7   5   3   1   hardcover

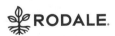

For Timmy
You boost me big time, honey. Love you.
and
To my dearly missed and loved friend and colleague
Rishi Angras (1977–2015)

CONTENTS

FROM ME TO YOU: WHY I WROTE THIS BOOK   I

INTRODUCTION: THE HORMONE BOOST AND YOU   7

PART ONE: THE FAT-LOSS SIX

1: Fat-Loss Hormone #1: Thyroid Hormone   23
   – Your Metabolic Master

2: Fat-Loss Hormone #2: Accelerate with Adrenaline   42

3: Fat-Loss Hormone #3: The Androgenic Hormones   50
   – DHEA and Testosterone

4: Fat-Loss Hormone #4: Growth Hormone and Acetylcholine   65
   – Hormones of Strength and Rejuvenation

5: Fat-Loss Hormone #5: Any Way You Add It Up,   79
Adiponectin Subtracts Fat

6: Fat-Loss Hormone #6: Go, Go, Glucagon!   93

7: Brain Boost: Happy, Mentally Sharp and Craving-Free   106
   – Dopamine, Serotonin and Melatonin

PART TWO: GET PREPPED

8: Three-Step Home Prep   133

9: Four-Step Body Prep   159

PART THREE: THE HORMONE BOOST ACTION PLAN

10: The Hormone Boost Nutrition Plan   185

11: The Hormone Boost Supplement Plan   207

12: The Hormone Boost Workout   219

PART FOUR: FOOD LISTS, SHOPPING LISTS AND RECIPES

13: Permitted Foods and Grocery Lists   245

14: The Recipes   267

APPENDIX: THE HORMONE BOOST SUCCESS TRACKER   313

RESOURCES   320

ACKNOWLEDGMENTS   323

GENERAL INDEX   325

RECIPE INDEX   335

ABOUT THE AUTHOR   343

FROM ME TO YOU:
WHY I WROTE THIS BOOK

*It's time to say goodbye, but I think goodbyes are sad and
I'd much rather say hello. Hello to a new adventure.*

ERNIE HARWELL,

sportscaster for 55 years,

42 of them with the Detroit Tigers

In my early twenties, just a few months after my graduation from
university in 1993, I arrived home one day from my summer job in
tears and feeling overwhelmed. I couldn't think. My head was buzz-
ing with confusion. I felt weak and feverish. I couldn't understand
people when they spoke to me. I couldn't seem to process information fast enough to make sense of anything. I thought I was going
crazy and was certain I had a serious neurological disease.

I had a friend take me to the emergency room, where the doctors found I indeed had a fever, along with severe anemia. They
told me to take some iron and to go home and rest, which was
about all I was capable of. I would wake up feeling okay, but within
minutes the confusion and fogginess in my head would return.
Even in this state, I began to realize something had been off for
months. I had needed so much sleep—over 16 hours a day—and
was too tired to go to the gym, even though I was an exercise

fanatic. I was gaining weight—almost 25 pounds. My periods were irregular and I was losing fistfuls of hair. I had chalked it all up to the stress of finishing school and ending a relationship with my boyfriend at the time.

Luckily the emergency room doctor investigated further into why I was so anemic and tested my blood (TSH level) to rule out hypothyroidism. Days later, I received a call letting me know my TSH was over 25, when a normal level is considered to be less than 4.7 and an optimal level is less than 2. I was severely hypothyroid, with extremely low iron levels and a low red-blood-cell count. Confusion was overcoming me because my brain function was slowing down along with the rest of me. I started taking thyroid medication immediately. Within a week I felt like a completely different person, and I continue to take thyroid medication today.

Looking back, I know I had the telltale symptoms of hypothyroidism as early as age 13. I remember waking up with my pillow covered in my hair and being taken to dermatologists for hair loss, but nothing those doctors proposed ever helped. I remember feeling tired all the time and having horrible menstrual issues, including pain, cramping and irregular cycles. I always had belly fat and would never wear a two-piece bathing suit. Now I know my disease was missed because I seemed to be slim. Because my weight appeared "normal," my doctors did not think of looking for hypothyroidism, a condition commonly found in noticeably overweight people.

Move on to 2000 and entering my thirties. After finishing four years of training, I began my practice as a naturopathic doctor. Yet somehow, and in direct contrast to my new wellness profession, I developed an addiction to cookies and muffins because I craved them so badly. And after the quest for these sugary treats, it was always followed by fighting to stay awake and a "carb coma." At the same time, my periods were becoming more irregular, my breasts were shrinking, my waist was getting wider and I was losing hair—again.

On a professional hunch, I underwent a thorough investigation involving blood work and ultrasounds. My suspicions were confirmed—I had polycystic ovarian syndrome (PCOS). PCOS is a condition characterized by irregular periods, hair loss, infertility, acne and weight gain; it's also linked to infertility and an increased risk of breast cancer and diabetes. So I now had not one but two metabolic diseases. Since PCOS is associated with insulin resistance, the underlying cause of type 2 diabetes, insulin-sensitizing medications such as metformin are regularly prescribed to treat it. And I was definitely insulin resistant. Besides the high insulin levels detected by my blood work, my cravings, constant hunger, fatigue after eating and fat gain around my abdomen were obvious signs.

Fast forward to today and my forties. So far this decade is proving to be interesting and dynamic as the demands on me naturally continue to evolve, compounded with the responsibility of a new role within my family. Career pressures, a tax audit, overseeing my business, personal worries, plus the commitment (as well as the honor and pleasure) of managing my mom's health-care needs, form past and present contributing factors to my stress and high cortisol levels. Thank goodness I possess the ability and know-how to effectively tackle the impact of these hormonal changes with diet, supplements and necessary adjustments to my thyroid prescription (I still continue to take thyroid medication that provides T4, but in the past few years I have required added compounded T3 to improve my thyroid profile).

As trying as they are, I am grateful for my experiences of hormonal concerns. Combined with years of clinical practice, they have allowed me to gain a much clearer view of the *real* big picture. Which brings me to a new topic of discussion—my friend in her forties, who I think of as the target audience for this book. She's healthier, in some ways, than she's ever been: She stopped smoking four years ago, eats an almost vegetarian diet with lots of the right proteins and whole grains, watches her alcohol intake and tries to get some form of exercise every day (walking, strength training or yoga). But she feels like she's in a bit of a rut. "It's not that there's any one thing wrong," she said in a recent conversation. "It's more that I think things really could be better." You might be feeling this way too—thinking about areas in your life that might be "okay" but could be "better." We live in an all-or-nothing world. Everything is *amazing* or *terrible.* We're multitasking on the go or hiding in bed from it all. Why is the idea that we're actually doing okay, slowly and incrementally achieving successes, so hard to hold on to? Why can't we be content with our lives while at the same time acknowledging that there's room to improve them? Accepting that we are on the right path—and being open to an even better experience while we're on it—doesn't really seem to have a place in our conversations about health and lifestyle. I think it should.

As a specialist in hormonal health, I've practiced for 15-plus years and have personally managed my own hormonal imbalances for over twenty. So I have a bit of experience in this subject. Hormonal imbalances have been the subject of my research for three bestselling books, and I've listened to thousands of cases in my clinical practice. But it was this conversation with my forty-year-old friend that got me thinking: Why was I, and why were most other specialists in this area, primarily focused on identifying *problems*? Why not shift our focus to the things that we are doing right, right now, so we can optimize them and achieve our desired outcomes?

So often we focus on what's wrong in our lives, and we tend to adopt an all-or-nothing approach to these things. If we have one night of overindulgence (alcohol, junk food, whatever your vice), we swear we're never going to touch it again. What if we spent our time instead on what we are happy with, and simply said, "More of this, please!" Focusing on what we want—more energy, a stronger memory or a faster metabolism, for example—allows us to examine our current practices for things that already support those goals. Not only does that help fix the problems of the past as a natural consequence, it also gives us the greatest chance of success. When we move from being problem-oriented to being outcome-oriented, we can tap into our best selves.

A Whole New Perspective

This shift from *current problem* to *desired outcome* was a big change for me, and exploring it led naturally to the field of positive psychology. This science of the positive in human life uses the same scientific tools as clinical psychology but has different central concerns: What makes us happy, what helps us flourish and what increases our well-being, creativity and optimism? It's the perfect framework—and starting point—for this book.

Introduced by psychologist, educator and author Martin Seligman, positive psychology lets go of the disease model, which tends to focus on the negative aspects of mental health—anxiety, depression and other mental illness—and turns instead to a *well-being* model. When we focus on well-being, we spend our time thinking about what makes life worth living, how we can make our daily lives, in my friend's word, "better." By examining the optimal ways in which we function, positive psychology aims to discover and promote the factors that allow individuals and communities to thrive.

And so, out of a conversation with a good friend, a quest for a new way of thinking, and a lot of new research, *The Hormone Boost* was born. It's not about overhauling your life in one day, one week or even one month. It's not going to tell you that all of your choices are terrible, and it won't try to sell you a magical plan that will "fix" everything. Instead, it will encourage you to recognize where you are, pinpoint what you want to improve, and consider how you can thrive. In other words, it's about giving you a boost—regardless of where you are in your health journey. This program will help you thrive by optimizing your hormonal health—and *fast*! The benefits for your hormones start right away, with whichever action you choose to undertake first, whether it is a Hormone

Boost meal, a good night's rest, a supplement, a workout or more.

Boost is such a great word for what's ahead. My goal is to give you a boost in the best sense of the word: to help you improve, gain confidence, achieve success—to lift you up and provide that extra help needed so you can get somewhere you can't quite reach on your own. But a boost can mean other things too, like positive and public dialogue; we often get "signal boosts" online when friends or colleagues are trying to spread the word about something important, something worth our time. And a boost can also refer to tapping into a power source for a fresh start, like boosting a car engine. In all its forms, then, a boost is what comes from collaboration focused on improvement.

Remember that positive psychology emphasis on thriving communities? Most of us crave community; in fact, part of our optimal human functioning involves healthy communities and partnerships. My friend told me just the other day, after having read through an earlier draft of this book, that she's now sharing the principles presented here with her partner—and together they've made tangible changes toward that better life she was craving. There is nothing that thrills me more than knowing that this work inspires people to give themselves and others a boost. And that's precisely what this book is designed to do for you. Are you ready to give it a go?

THE HORMONE BOOST AND YOU

The good life is a process, not a state of being.

CARL ROGERS,
American psychologist, known for the "person-centered approach"

The conversation that started me down the Hormone Boost path made me realize how many people these days fit into a "just okay" mold—a way of existing from day to day that isn't awful but sure isn't great, either. Perhaps you feel the same way. When I stopped and really thought about it, I realized this shouldn't have come as a surprise. In my practice, I hear from people all the time—all day, every day, in fact—about what they want more of, or what they want to improve. There's a lot of common ground in these discussions, and chances are good that you've had the same thoughts from time to time (or maybe more often). This, then, is where we begin: with the biggest and most important areas in need of a boost.

How 'bout a Boost of These . . .

While there is an almost endless supply of areas in our daily lives that can be improved, the following seven are the ones that crop up most often in the discussions I've had about well-being.

Energy

Regular sleep and regular exercise combined with a thoughtful diet should be sufficient to give anyone the energy they need for a busy life. The thing is, if we're not getting the right kinds of sleep, practicing the right exercises or eating the right foods, we can wreak havoc on our energy levels without even knowing it. If part of how you're managing your days right now requires the assistance of regular caffeine intake, high-sugar foods, or an afternoon nap, you'll be interested in *The Hormone Boost*'s plan to power up your energy by targeting the specific hormones and habits that affect it most intensely.

Strength

Being strong isn't just about being able to open the pickle jar without special implements or assistance. It's also about creating the optimum conditions for your body to take care of itself and move freely through the world. Whatever your limitations are (in terms of health, work or mobility), a stronger body will improve your energy and quality of life. It can even make sitting at a desk for several hours more manageable, and allow you to burn more fat while doing it! Strong bodies also age more gracefully and recover from illness and injury more quickly. We're not able to get any younger, but we can *always* get stronger. The Hormone Boost plan will show you how.

Memory

We might not notice our memory gaps in this always connected ultra-digital world. Can't remember a celebrity's name? You can IMDB it. Worried about forgetting a new contact's number? Put it in your smartphone. Never before have we had so many devices stand in for memory. As a result, unsurprisingly, our memories are not as strong as they used to be. (I once nearly drove myself crazy trying to remember an actor's name—and I refused to look it up online. It took me three days but I trusted that her name was in there, and sure enough, it was: Reese Witherspoon. *Boom.*) It's impractical to disengage completely from all of your devices and external reminders, but you can give your memory a genuine boost by attending to the hormones that give it strength and longevity. Quicker, more intense memory recall is part of a strong, active brain—and it supports your mental acuity.

Metabolism

It's hard to be healthy and energetic and fit without metabolic support. As I mentioned previously, I went through an intense struggle with my metabolism after graduating from university, and again six years later, after naturopathic medical school. During both periods, my strict diet and rigorous exercise sessions failed to help me lose weight or keep it off. It was during those times that my hormonal health concerns forced me to realize that the formula *calories in – calories burned = weight loss* was by no means complete. Hormones are the body's powerhouse; the processes they drive sustain every aspect of health and fat-burning potential (a.k.a. metabolism). Boosting your metabolism means augmenting your capacity to generate and use energy—and that is naturally connected to your health, energy and fitness levels.

Confidence

Regardless of your size or style, you should be confident. Full stop. The people I am most drawn to are those who just seem *entirely comfortable with themselves*—people who own their worth, who wouldn't trade places with anyone. This is what I wish for all of my patients and friends, because it can make such a massive difference in every area of your life: professionally, personally (especially in intimate relationships), physically. Confidence walks with a straight back and long strides and a general peace with the world. Balancing your hormones, especially those discussed in this book, will allow you to generate confidence in your sense of surety and comfort with your body, your life and your relationships.

Immunity

The twenty-first century has brought with it an amazing number of quick fixes and surface shortcuts—and we rely on them to make our lives easier in countless ways. Too often, though, we don't stop and think about the challenges this reliance is creating. Take hand sanitizer. While effective in the immediate biological sense (e.g., after using the toilet), its prevalence is making it harder and harder for our bodies to build up their own immunities. Ditto for antibiotics, which, when overprescribed, compromise our ability to fight off seemingly minor viruses and bacteria. I'm not suggesting you swear off sanitizer entirely or avoid a doctor's prescription, but I invite you to explore what a hormonally boosted immune system can do. If the metabolism is the body's powerhouse, the immune system is the Neighborhood Watch: It monitors comings and goings and does its best to ensure you're safe. A hormone boost to the metabolism increases not only its efficacy but also your overall safety.

Mood

Boosting your mood has a more subtle impact, in some ways, than boosting your metabolism or immune system. A mood boost won't necessarily help you lose a few pounds or fend off the flu that's going around. But our moods are pervasive, and they have the power to change our perspective, our schedule and our interactions. Wake up in a bad mood? You might swear at the thought of hard-boiled eggs for breakfast and grab a croissant instead. Have an unexpectedly tense confrontation with a client or colleague? You might treat yourself to a beer as soon as you get in the door, to help unwind after that adrenaline-inducing conversation. When you're in a good mood, you are more patient (you'll walk home rather than jump in a cab), make better choices (cheerfully crunch that salad—and those abs!) and attract the good energies of others (that stranger you bumped into at the produce stand just happens to be a trainer at your local gym and invites you in for a free session). Boosting your mood will have a thousand small positive effects in every area of your life.

The Hormone Boost has been diligently researched and designed to boost every part of you. We'll explore each boost area and its corresponding hormones thoroughly, unpacking the science behind hormonal health and tracing the connections between what we do and how we feel. I'm also thrilled to be able to share with you some amazing successes from my practice; they demonstrate just how important hormonal health is in all areas of your life. And each chapter will leave you with my recommendations for boosting the hormones that are integral to powering up your body, your mind and your fat-loss efforts. Specifically, we're going to focus on a group of hormones I've come to think of as "the fat-loss six."

Not Just Another Fad

I know it can be a challenge to encounter a new idea or theory and not think of it as just the latest fad in a world designed to reel us in. I'm sure you've heard on social media, in the news and amongst your friends a hundred of the "best" new things to try in order to feel younger, smarter, more vibrant. It's hard, in our click-bait world, to think through new ideas without a healthy (and necessary!) dose of skepticism.

But through that really loud noise, some new theories and ways of thinking are, in fact, giving us more pertinent information about how we live and how we can thrive. A 2015 study on subjective age, for example, discovered that how old we feel has a lot more to do with our daily health, regular stressors and emotional affects than the years we've clocked. The study asked forty-three older adults, aged 60 to 93, to fill out daily questionnaires over the course of eight days. Researchers were interested in learning if "felt ages" fluctuate from day to day, and if daily changes in health, stressors and affects mirror those fluctuations.

What they discovered is intriguing. Differences in the partici-pants' "felt ages" were explained not by the passage of time but by the other variables: The average health problems, stress or negative affects they experienced on a particular day made them feel older than they felt on days when they did not experience them. Let me repeat that: *Average health problems, stress and negative emotional affects make you feel older than you actually are.*

If we flip this conclusion on its head, we come right back to the boost philosophy: We can focus on the choices and behaviors that make us healthy, unstressed and optimistic—and *do more of them.* That's why we're going to target specific fat-loss and well-being areas and the hormones that boost them. Not only will we be setting the ideal conditions for us to thrive, we will also likely feel younger, stronger and better. Anyone interested in turning that down?

The Joy of Six: Introducing the Fat-Loss Six

Ask anyone if they know a hormone that causes weight loss. Most people will mention the thyroid hormone. That's true, but did you know there are actually *six* hormones that impact fat loss? *The Hormone Boost* is your comprehensive guide to powering up the group I refer to as "the fat-loss six": thyroid hormones, adrenaline, glucagon, adiponectin, the androgenic hormones (DHEA and tes-tosterone) and the growth and rejuvenation hormones (growth hor-mone and acetylcholine). These super-performers help us get lean and strong in two key ways: They directly stimulate metabolism, or the breakdown of body-fat stores for energy, and they stimulate fat loss by supporting the growth of metabolically active muscle. In the next sections, I'll tell you how.

Thyroid Hormones (TSH, Free T3 and Free T4)

The masters of your metabolism, these hormones drive every sin-gle cell in your body. It all starts with TSH (thyroid-stimulating hormone). TSH, in turn, stimulates thyroxine (free T4), which is then converted to triiodothyronine (free T3). When all three are functioning properly and produced in the correct amounts, your metabolism is a fat-burning machine. And that's what we're aiming for!

Adrenaline

Also known as epinephrine, adrenaline is responsible for revving you up (think fight-or-flight response and all the physical effects it has on your body). This handy hormone allows the body to free up the fats and sugars it's stored so that we have that burst of energy we need when we really need it.

Glucagon

Think of glucagon as insulin's helpful opposite: Rather than lowering blood sugar by transporting glucose from the bloodstream (and into liver, muscle and fat cells) for storage as glycogen or fat, glucagon *raises* blood sugar by breaking down the fat and glycogen that were stored. We can tap into this awesome hormone through exercising, consuming protein, or experiencing a dip in blood sugar. (Don't worry, we'll fully review good carb/bad carb, glycemic index/glycemic load details in Chapter 6.)

Adiponectin

Adiponectin isn't nearly as well known as the previous three hormones—and that's really too bad. This fantastic hormone is produced in and sent out from your fat cells, but it's also got a direct and reciprocal relationship with them, which means that although it's produced by your fat cells, it actually *helps burn up fat*! Even better, the higher your adiponectin levels, the higher your energy and caloric expenditure. And because it increases insulin sensitivity, it also improves glucose tolerance and inhibits inflammation.

The Androgenic Hormones (DHEA and Testosterone)

Let's talk about sex, baby! And by that I mean sex hormones. DHEA (dehydroepiandrosterone—yes, that's a real word, and a really important hormone) comes from the adrenal glands and leads the charge for estrogen and testosterone. A DHEA boost is definitely part of your hormonal powering up because of its ability to support metabolically active muscle growth. Muscle growth is key to fat loss, so attending to DHEA is part of this program. DHEA will support your immune system, improve tissue repair and sleep and neutralize the impact of cortisol (the stress hormone), among a host of other benefits. And testosterone? It's almost impossible to build muscle mass without enough of this hormone—for both men and women—and testosterone is also connected to improvements in libido, bone density, strength, motivation, memory, fat burning and skin tone. Boosting this dynamic duo is a huge part of realizing your health and vitality goals.

The Growth and Rejuvenation Hormones (Growth Hormone and Acetylcholine)

It's impossible to discuss fat loss and muscle growth without touching on growth hormone and acetylcholine. Released during deep sleep, growth hormone is almost magical in its ability to repair tissue and build muscle. Its regenerative powers can make a huge difference in your fat-loss and muscle-growth goals. And when it comes to communicating with muscles to encourage their movement, coordination and tone, you need the right amounts of acetylcholine. Because we use up this hormone when we exercise, boosting its levels is imperative for maintaining strong, healthy and metabolically-active muscle.

What an amazing collection of health benefits a boost of these six hormones can bring! But we're not done yet. No boost is complete without getting the brain involved. And for that, we turn to a trio of hormones that control your appetite, mood and sleep patterns, as well as perform other functions that fuel fat loss.

Serotonin, Melatonin and Dopamine

Serotonin, melatonin and dopamine are hormones and neuro-transmitters (communication systems between the brain and the body), which make them effective mood boosters. They also regulate sleep habits and food cravings and manage concentration, weight and digestion. You've likely heard about melatonin before—that nightly boost that invites growth hormone to work its magic. Melatonin influences nervous system function, but it's a delicate hormone; it requires the right conditions (full darkness, coolness and absence of caffeine, alcohol and smoke) in order to be effective. Adequate amounts of serotonin and dopamine help regulate your appetite and sense of satiety, as well as stimulate brain activity and motivation. Appetite regulation is more complex than you might realize; it's not enough to simply will yourself to eat less. Your hormones are responding to all kinds of messages and conditions that could make even the most self-disciplined person head for the junk-food aisle.

Focusing on your hormonal health is obviously a big part of *The Hormone Boost*, but it's not the only key to success. You need to be ready and willing to accept new ways of thinking about your overall health, and to focus on some life changes that pave the way for a positive approach.

The TurnTash Method

Tidying up—it's all the rage right now, and for good reason. We have more stuff than we've ever had, and less space and time to properly use or enjoy it. It's no surprise, then, that a little book about how to tidy up and change your life has spawned a revolution (not to mention two follow-up books, including an illustrated "master class" on folding clothes and organizing drawers, and a daily journal!). I believe that a huge part of its success is its positive emphasis—rather than shaming us for keeping things we don't need, shouldn't have or were crazy to want in the first place, it asks us to consider all the objects in our home, individually, to see whether they *bring us joy.*

If the KonMari Method is followed carefully (and it is an exact, intentional process), you'll end up with fewer objects (paper, clothes, photos, knick-knacks, etc.) to deal with every day. More importantly, you'll also end up with more joy when you encounter the objects that remain—and more space to welcome new objects, experiences and relationships, along with new actions, habits and mindsets. Closets are uncluttered. Drawers are minimalistic and well organized. Bookshelves can breathe, and your floors have room for you to dance.

Imagine tapping in to this process as part of a new approach to your overall health, diet and exercise. What currently brings you joy on this front? What are you ready to let go of? What are you ready to try? Imagine your body free of toxins, your mind clear and focused. Your major systems (metabolic and otherwise) have the power to perform at their best, and your hormones are receiving the boost they need so you can dance into your best life. The joy at the heart of the KonMari Method is precisely like the boost at the heart of this book—it's all about choosing the foods and practices that give us the best hormonal health, and simply letting go of the rest.

The Hormone Boost Starts Here

I've said it before and I'll say it again: The body is a complex system, even in ideal conditions and with the best possible habits and practices in place. When you reach the point in your life where you're starting to reflect on what's working (thanks, positive psychology) and you're keen to prioritize what brings you joy (the TurnTash Method), you're ready for this book. In the pages that follow, I will give you the lift you need to reach your goals (and you're already so close!).

First, we'll spend some time getting to know the fat-loss six (and that helpful brain-boosting trio) a bit better. You'll learn why it's so important to give these particular hormones a helping hand. We'll explore the science behind the boost and learn about diet, exercise and lifestyle recommendations that can help you begin powering up now.

Then we'll follow up the science with some simple steps to prep the three most crucial areas in your home: your kitchen, bathroom and bedroom. Tidying up these areas so they're free of the products and conditions that disrupt hormones is integral to your hormonal health success. Not only will we remove what's harmful and unnecessary, we'll also boost each room's ideal state—your bedroom will be the perfect environment for sleep; your bathroom will be free of products that contain harmful chemicals and hormone disruptors; and your kitchen will serve as a mecca for healthy, hormonally-balanced meals.

From the external to the internal, we'll also explore simple steps that focus on your body. Three of its major organs—the skin, liver and digestive system—have a profound effect on all your hormones. We'll take the time to talk through restoring and optimizing their function before we embark on the positive action plans that comprise the nutrition, supplement and exercise strategies of *The Hormone Boost*.

Then we'll get to the part where theory becomes practice—with my Hormone Boost diet. Because this book focuses on the positive, we're going to skip the detox phase. (If that's an important first step for you, you can find instructions and support in *The Hormone Diet* and *The Supercharged Hormone Diet*.) What I've laid out for you here are simple daily rules with suggested tweaks to keep your metabolism guessing and your fat-loss six revving. I truly believe this is my simplest and most effective diet yet. It's been clear and easy to go over with my patients, and we're seeing results quickly—without hunger or cravings, and with a significant boost in energy and brain power. These effects are consistently reported in *four days*. Seriously. Within this plan, you will consume four meals per day, with the right amounts of protein, fat, carbs and fiber for you. And because I know from personal experience that focusing on positive changes works best with full support, I have provided simple lists that will help you create your own Hormone Boost meals, salads and smoothies. There are also more than 50 tried-and-treasured recipes, if you're in need of some inspiration.

Next we'll review a few essential supplements that ideally go hand-in-hand with your Hormone Boost meals (probiotics, vitamin D, omega, vitamins E and C, and the minerals zinc and magnesium). While supplement suggestions are included in each of the fat-loss-six chapters, Chapter 11 is where you'll get the in-depth information that will help you decide which supplements are right for you, and how to take them safely. I've included the rationale behind each supplement, because I believe it's important to fully understand how and why they work. For now, you can think of them as accelerators for the fat-loss six: They boost and enable hormone activity. Many of these nutrients also support the organs that impact your hormones, especially your skin and digestive system.

Finally we hit the sweet spot of the Hormone Boost—the perfect workout to power up your fat-loss six. Perfect? Absolutely! It's the result of research and experience, and I use it myself, so I can vouch for its effectiveness. An incredible combo of walking (or one to two short interval cardio sessions), yoga and strength training, this workout plan gets you moving, stretching and building muscle. The strength-training workouts are based on German Body Composition Training—a style that is one of the few methods *proven* to simultaneously boost fat loss and muscle growth. It creates the perfect positive hormonal response we all should be striving for. It's short and tough, but its results are indisputable.

And throughout the book, I'll share with you stories of success taken from my own practice. It's inspiring to see so many men and women who have used the Hormone Boost program and achieved such positive results. If you ever have a moment of doubt or a day when you're just not "feeling it," these real-life examples will be just what you need to stay on track.

And Now . . .

I am genuinely excited about the positive, joy-filled journey you're about to take. You *will* have fun and feel amazing! And I want to remind you, the philosophy of this book is about acceptance and improvement, being open to new ways of thinking about what you eat and how you move while retaining the habits and practices that are currently working for you. It's also about collaboration—your interest and commitment combined with my expertise and planning. Together, we can get you where you want to go.

A HORMONE BOOST REAL-LIFE SUCCESS STORY

THE CLIENT: Marlene W.

DETAILS: Female, 43

**BODY COMPOSITION RESULTS (FROM SCALE AND BODY FAT/
MUSCLE MASS VIA BIO-IMPEDANCE TESTING)**

MEASUREMENT	BEFORE	AFTER	TOTAL LOSS/GAIN
Weight (lb.)	157.8	130	(−)27.8
Lean Body Mass (lb.)	104.1	102.7	(−) 1.4
Fat Mass (lb.)	53.7	29.3	(−) 24.4
Basal Metabolic Rate (calories/day)	1,473 calories	1,437 calories	(−) 36

I have loved working with Marlene from day one (October 29, 2014) and actually had the pleasure of seeing her while I was completing the work on this book (in December 2015). She has an incredible commitment to her health and to learning. She's stuck with the supplements, diet and strength training perfectly—and her results prove it.

Marlene is a picture-perfect Hormone Boost transformation. She lost almost 25 pounds of fat and a negligible amount of muscle. After all of her weight loss, she ended up with the ideal amount of muscle for her frame. Her sleep, energy and skin have improved. And the abdominal bloating she experienced also cleared up.

PART ONE

THE FAT-LOSS SIX

You've got to get up every morning with determination
if you're going to go to bed with satisfaction.

GEORGE LORIMER,
American journalist and author, best known
as editor of the *Saturday Evening Post*

CHAPTER 1

FAT-LOSS HORMONE #1:
THYROID HORMONE
YOUR METABOLIC MASTER

Ability is what you're capable of doing. Motivation determines what you do. Attitude determines how well you do it.

LOU HOLTZ,
former American football player and coach

Let's begin *The Hormone Boost* by discussing your metabolic master: the thyroid hormones, which influence every single cell in your body—every tissue, every organ. Sounds impressive, right? It is. In fact, it was a deficiency of thyroid hormone decades ago that started my experience with, and work on, hormone health. I guess you could say that I owe my thyroid a thing or two!

Thyroid Basics

Your thyroid is situated in the front of your neck, just below your Adam's apple. It's a butterfly-shaped gland, the "wings" of which extend to either side of your windpipe. It's not all that big, but it produces multiple, and powerful, hormones. Together, these hormones regulate our metabolism and organ function, directly affecting almost every bodily system and function: heart rate, cholesterol levels, weight, energy, muscle contraction and relaxation, skin and hair texture, bowel function, fertility, menstrual regularity, memory, mood and more. It is well documented that normal levels of thyroid hormone are also essential to the development of the fetal and neonatal brain.

Thyroid hormones increase the heart's rate and workload by increasing the number and force of heart contractions. This, along with the naturally dilating effects of thyroid hormones on blood vessels, helps to improve blood flow to many organs. Thyroid hormones are essential for the proper development of all the body's cells. They allow the body to become more sensitive to all other hormones, in turn making them more effective. Finally, our reproductive system function and physiology is dependent on sufficient levels of thyroid hormone. (For instance, I usually suspect low thyroid hormone, or low estrogen, when a patient's menstrual cycle is longer than 30 days.)

The Thyroid–Metabolism Connection

Many years of clinical studies and research have revealed the complex relationship between thyroid disease, body weight and metabolism. Thyroid hormone regulates the metabolism in both animals and humans. Metabolism is determined by measuring the amount of oxygen used by the body over a specific period of time. If the measurement is taken at rest, it is known as the basal metabolic rate (BMR). Indeed, BMR measurement was one of the earliest tests used to assess a patient's thyroid status. Patients whose thyroid glands were underperforming were found to have low BMRs, and those with overactive thyroid glands had high BMRs (keep in mind that a low BMR usually equates to trouble dropping extra pounds).

Thyroid hormones also regulate the body's ability to impact protein, fat and carbohydrate metabolism, thereby boosting protein synthesis and, ultimately, energy, while increasing the breakdown of stored carbohydrates. This effect is mediated by beta adrenergic receptors (which help us burn fat). By acting on beta adrenergic receptors, certain thyroid hormones can increase heart and pulse rates. They can also increase the burn rate of body fat stores; specifically, they help to break down cholesterol and lower low-density lipoprotein (LDL)—which is also why many people with low or suboptimal thyroid hormones tend to experience an increase in cholesterol. All of these effects combined allow the body to burn more calories and use them more efficiently, which is our goal when it comes to being healthy and fit. For this reason, thyroid hormones have commonly been used as fat-loss drugs.

Meet the Thyroid Hormones

TSH (Thyroid-Stimulating Hormone)

TSH is produced by the pituitary gland under direction from the hypothalamus. Elevated levels of TSH suggest that the thyroid gland is failing to respond properly to this signal from the pituitary that tells it to make more hormones. TSH is measured on a scale of 0.35 to 5 for most laboratory sources. My clinical experience, however, suggests that the optimal level for TSH is less than 2, and in some cases, even closer to 1.

Free T4

T4 (thyroxine) is the thyroid hormone produced directly by the thyroid gland in response to stimulation from TSH. It is made up of iodine and the amino acid tyrosine. The optimal value for T4 is the middle to upper range of the lab's normal results (which can vary from lab to lab).

Free T3

T4 is converted to T3 (triiodothyronine) in the cells of the body. In fact, T3 directly influences the metabolism of every single cell, tissue and organ in the body. The optimal measurement for free T3 is like T4—a value toward the high end of the lab's normal reference range (again, this can vary).

Reverse T3

Reverse triiodothyronine (rT3) differs from T3 in the positions of the iodine atoms attached to the aromatic rings. The majority of rT3 found in blood circulation is formed by the removal of an iodine atom from T4 (thyroxine). rT3 is believed to be metabolically inactive.

The levels of T3 and T4 in the body act as negative feedback mechanisms that stop the production of thyroid hormone until it's needed again. This also means that low levels of T3 and T4 will increase TSH production, which is indicative of low thyroid hormones or hypothyroidism.

The Production and Activation of Thyroid Hormone

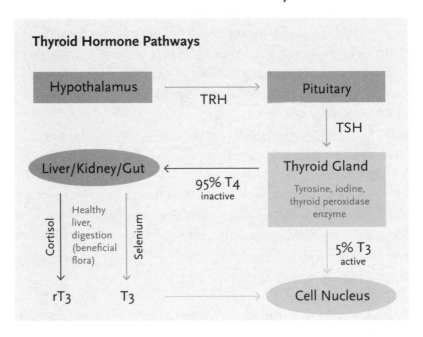

In order for your thyroid to work properly—produce the right amounts and types of hormones—a lot of things have to go right. In essence, proper thyroid hormone metabolism and activation require several other glands and systems to work properly. These include the pituitary gland, the liver, the digestive system and the adrenals. Your thyroid gland also relies on key nutrients for thyroid hormone to be manufactured and utilized properly. The diagram on page 26 shows just how complex and interconnected this process can be. Most important:

- Your pituitary gland needs to make TSH properly.
- Proper enzyme (thyroid-peroxidase) activity, iodine uptake and sufficient levels of tyrosine are all needed within the thyroid to make thyroid hormones (primarily T4).
- Conversion of T4 to T3 thyroid hormone and activation must take place in the liver, digestive system (healthy bacteria levels influence this) and kidneys. Selenium is also needed for the healthy production of T3.
- To prevent excess rT3 (which can bind to T3 receptor sites but fail to promote its beneficial metabolic effects), cortisol needs to be balanced. Both adrenal gland function and stress levels, therefore, impact thyroid hormone production and activation.
- Last, effective metabolic and other natural activities of the T3 have to occur in the cells of the body (after binding to receptors).

Your body is a complex system, and all of these moving pieces help to explain why a comprehensive strategy produces superior outcomes when striving for a thyroid boost, especially for those with thyroid hormone–related issues.

Low Thyroid: A Common Concern with Serious Consequences

Low thyroid (also referred to as sluggish thyroid, thyroid deficiency or subclinical hypothyroidism) means that your thyroid gland is producing fewer thyroid hormones than your body needs. Because the thyroid gland is a vital link in the endocrine system, even a small decline in the output of thyroid hormone, if sustained over an extended period of time, can have profound consequences for health and longevity. And, it turns out, lower thyroid activity is definitely tied to weight gain. An April 2008 study out of New York reported that middle-aged adults with mildly underactive thyroid gland activity (that is, on the low side of normal) may be prone to weight gain. The study included 2,407 men and women who were an average of 48 years old when the study began. Among its findings:

- In women, the average weight for those with slightly elevated levels of TSH was 142 pounds, versus 155 for those with the highest TSH levels; women with the highest TSH levels gained an average of 9.3 pounds more than women with the lowest TSH levels.
- In men, the average weight was 182 pounds in participants with the lowest TSH and 189 pounds in those with higher levels. The average weight gain in men with the highest TSH levels, compared to those with the lowest levels, was 4.2 pounds greater.

Low thyroid most often affects women over forty, but men and even teenagers can also have reduced thyroid function, especially if it runs in the family (my husband, Tim, swears he "caught" his thyroid condition from me—even though both his mother and his sister have been diagnosed with hypothyroidism and take prescription medications to manage it!). According to some estimates, as many as 15 to 20 percent of women over the age of sixty may have subclinical hypothyroidism. This means that they would benefit from thyroid supplementation, even though most conventional doctors would insist, based on standard laboratory test results, that there was no need for treatment. Every year, a substantial percentage of these women develop symptoms (such as fatigue, hair loss, constipation, feeling cold, weight gain or inability to lose), some of which may contribute to shortened life expectancy. Case in point: Heart disease is the number one killer of women. As we've seen, when thyroid hormones are suboptimal, cholesterol can rise. It is incredibly important, then, for thyroid hormones to be—and stay—optimized. Peri- and post-menopausal women should pay especially close attention to their thyroid—up to 20 percent of this population develop issues with suboptimal thyroid, which impacts cardiovascular health at a life stage that already includes the risk of heart disease.

Despite this reality, age-related thyroid decline remains underdiagnosed by many doctors, largely because they are not generally trained to look for it. It's not uncommon for physicians to rely more on laboratory results than the symptoms a patient may present. Also, many doctors—and their patients—seem willing to accept that these symptoms are normal signs of aging and fail to consider that something can be done. As doctors, we must consider the optimal range for thyroid and treat the patient, not the blood work. Being tired and lethargic and gaining weight is never normal!

A New Option for Underactive Thyroid?

For years, the treatment of underactive thyroid conditions has been the same: replacement of the T4 hormone, with the assumption that it will be converted to T3 in the body's tissues. But according to results reported in January 2015 from researchers at the University of North Carolina, adding T3 to the standard T4 treatment can boost mood and mental function.

Many patients who have lost their thyroid gland to cancer, surgery or injuries report feeling less mentally sharp, and they note that their sense of well-being, energy, memory and various other facets of their brain function have declined. Of the patients who received a combination of T3 and T4, all but two fared better in terms of memory, mood, concentration, depression, energy and other characteristics than their counterparts undergoing traditional therapy. When asked at the end of the study which treatment they preferred, twenty of the thirty-three participants chose the combined therapy.

I'm not surprised by these results. I take this combination of hormones myself, and often recommend a prescription of Eltroxin (T4) combined with Armour Thyroid (which provides T4 and T3 and has increased T3 in my patients' blood work) or compounded T3 for patients to keep both T3 and T4 in the optimal range. I've found that using Armour alone doesn't support enough T4. If you want to make this switch, it's best to titer your doses of the two slowly and test TSH, free T3 and free T4 every four weeks until the optimal range is reached.

Optimum Thyroid Levels for Pregnancy

Another important area in which we must stop relying on a laboratory's definition of "normal" is thyroid levels during pregnancy. There are large differences in normal thyroid function lab reference ranges among pregnant women. The importance of using correct reference intervals, however, is underlined by the fact that even small, subclinical variations in thyroid function have been associated with detrimental pregnancy outcomes, including low birth weight and pregnancy loss.

That means it's time for change; we need to give historical definitions of "normal" the boot and start relying instead on each woman's own pregnancy-specific reference intervals. During pregnancy, profound changes in thyroid physiology occur, resulting in different TSH and free T4 reference ranges compared to non-pregnant women. International guidelines recommend calculating trimester- and assay-specific reference intervals per trimester. If these reference intervals are unavailable, TSH reference intervals of 0.1 to 2.5 mU/L for the first trimester and 0.2 to 3.0 mU/L for the second trimester are recommended.

How Thyroid Hormone Works for You

So now you know all about the thyroid and how, when working properly, it can help you achieve optimal health by exerting an influence on every cell in your body. Now let's dive into how a properly functioning thyroid can work for you—every day—on the Hormone Boost plan.

Mood Boost

If you're looking for a mood boost, look no further than T3. In fact, I once consulted with a psychiatrist who informed me that thyroid drugs were used to treat depression before the invention of the selective serotonin reuptake inhibitor (SSRI) medications most commonly used today. T3's positive influence on depression comes from its specific activity within the brain; it increases the production of certain neurotransmitters, especially serotonin. According to these studies, however, it is not all-or-nothing—the positive effect of T3 on serotonin makes it a valuable recommendation for depression in some cases when used alone, and also when used in conjunction with SSRIs, and for the treatment of drug-resistant and recurring depression and bipolar disorders.

Brain Boost (Especially for Menopausal Women)

Recently, a group of 383 women took part in a study to assess cognitive function and thyroid status. The inclusion criteria were a minimum of two years since the last menstruation and no signs of dementia. A computerized battery of Central Nervous System Vital Signs tests was used to diagnose cognitive functions. The results, published in the *Indian Journal of Endocrinology and Metabolism* (May–June 2015), found that a higher TSH level (which, remember, means lower levels of thyroid hormone) was associated with decreases in memory, reaction time and verbal memory. Free T4 was positively correlated with faster reflex and response times. Even a modest reduction in TSH—a likely effect of following the nutrition plan and supplements in *The Hormone Boost*, by the way—is vital for enhancing cognitive function, especially in post-menopausal women.

Digestion Boost

Not only do you get a metabolic, mood and cognitive boost from thyroid hormone, it gives your digestion a boost too. For proper thyroid function, the T4 in your body must be converted into its active T3 form, which is partly done in the gastrointestinal tract. In order for this conversion to happen, the GI tract needs healthy colonies of beneficial bacteria. An imbalance in the good-to-bad bacteria ratio in the GI tract (dysbiosis) can lead to low thyroid function. This explains why so many patients with thyroid hormone imbalance also have digestive problems, and why digestive issues sometimes occur even in the presence of normal thyroid blood chemistry panels.

Chronic constipation is associated with *hypo*thyroidism, while diarrhea or frequent bowel movements are linked with higher thyroid hormone levels (*hyper*thyroidism). In the case of hyperthyroidism, the body's metabolism is essentially stuck in high gear and burning up body tissues much too rapidly. As a consequence, those with hyperthyroidism will feel hot and experience rapid heart rate, weight loss (or weight gain, if they eat a lot more because of increased appetite), irritability, insomnia, shakiness and digestive symptoms. Extreme energy states (hyper or fatigued) are very common as well.

These digestive symptoms are partly the result of an altered metabolism, but they can also be created by faulty digestion, which begins in the stomach. Hypothyroidism can reduce the production of stomach acid through its effect on the hormone gastrin. When too little gastrin is produced, the amount of stomach acid (HCl) is reduced. Bloating, gastroesophageal reflux disorder (GERD), heartburn, intestinal inflammation, decreased food digestion and more can result from the lack of normal HCl levels. To find out where your HCl levels are, I recommend completing the HCL Challenge. You can find the instructions in the "Book Extras" section for *The Hormone Diet* and *The Supercharged Hormone Diet* on www.drnatashaturner.com.

Food allergies are consistently seen in those with thyroid problems—no surprise, given the influence of thyroid hormones on digestion, transit time and stomach acid. Beyond gluten sensitivity, which most people are aware of, there are other food allergens for which patients will test positive. When I say "test positive," I'm referring to the results of a blood test that measures IgG antibodies for between 120 and 200 foods. (IgG antibodies are delayed reactions to specific food sensitivities, as compared to IgE-mediated reactions, which are immediate and can be anaphylactic.) Although results may vary greatly from one patient to the next, the most common food sensitivities include soy, eggs, wheat, citrus, cow's milk, cow's-milk cheese, cow's-milk yogurt and yeast.

In addition, there is another mechanism in the GI tract that can lead to low thyroid function. Your digestive tract is lined with lymph (immune) tissue known as GALT (gut-associated lymphoid tissue). Stress to the GALT can be caused by food sensitivities, undigested proteins, leaky gut, and infections from bacteria, yeast or parasites. These GALT afflictions can cause a major stress response, which raises your adrenal glands' production of cortisol. Cortisol, in turn, will cause a shift in thyroid hormone metabolism—increasing rT3 and causing an imbalance. Chronic cortisol elevation from stress will suppress the immune system in the GI tract, which can lead to dysbiosis, parasites, yeast and leaky gut—creating a vicious cycle that further disrupts thyroid function.

For all of these reasons, a healthy and balanced GI tract is extremely important in optimizing thyroid hormones and function. I have seen many patients whose thyroid function normalized after simply treating imbalances in the GI tract. In fact, if you have not done so already, I recommend completing the first three weeks of my 6-week

Supercharged Hormone Diet before starting your Hormone Boost plan. It will optimize digestion, restore HCl levels (if needed) and guide you through the process of identifying your food sensitivities. This will set you up for success with the Hormone Boost plan.

Heart Health Boost

Elevated cholesterol levels in the blood are indisputably associated with atherosclerosis and the risk of cardiovascular disease. Poorly managed hypothyroid patients, and those of us with suboptimal thyroid hormone activity, are at risk of high cholesterol. However, cholesterol is not the only indicator for cardiovascular risk. People with elevated levels of the amino acid homocysteine in their blood are also at risk for atherosclerosis and cardiovascular disease.

Some researchers believe that elevated homocysteine levels may be as much—or even more—of a risk factor than high cholesterol; I have seen it cause heart disease even when the cholesterol levels were normal. We now know that low thyroid can lead to high homocysteine levels. In a study from the *International Journal of Obesity and Related Metabolic Disorders* (June 2000), patients who'd had their thyroid gland completely removed and had stopped thyroid hormone supplementation were periodically tested for blood homocysteine and cholesterol, both of which were found to be increasing. When thyroid supplementation was reinstated, however, both of these substances were reduced to the patients' normal levels within four to six weeks.

So how does one go about lowering homocysteine levels? We need to consume foods and supplements high in the B vitamins: folic acid, B_6 and B_{12}. Clear Detox–Hormonal Health contains many of these ingredients and is recommended as part of your Hormone Boost supplement plan. Beyond this, though, I recommend using a combination of whole thyroid extract or supplements to boost thyroid function—likely the best way to combat elevated homocysteine levels and thereby reduce the risk of heart disease.

Weight-Loss Boost

When the body's production of thyroid hormone falls, the metabolic rate falls with it. In this regard, the amount of circulating T3 is actually more important than the amount of circulating T4. Because of the lowered metabolic rate, low thyroid function means difficulty in reducing body weight. When overweight individuals adopt healthy, low-caloric diets and take up regular exercise but still cannot shed weight, the most likely reason is a low metabolic rate caused by suboptimal or low T3 levels. Even a 10 percent reduction in metabolic rate can make weight loss very difficult. Available clinical data suggests, however, that most people who find it difficult to lose weight have a 15 to 40 percent reduction in metabolic rate.

If you suspect you are in this group, the Hormone Boost plan—especially the T3 boost it offers—could be your scientific remedy for losing weight. When boosting T3 for fat loss, the aim is to increase the levels of T3 to the edge of the upper limit while not stepping over and setting off hyperthyroidism. This plan is specifically designed to enhance your thyroid hormone without the risk of overstimulation.

Remember, T3's ability to prompt weight loss does not really depend on adopting a low-caloric diet. In fact, the usual response to a low-carbohydrate diet is a *reduction* in your metabolic rate. This is why a "cheat meal" once a week and a plan to optimize T3 will keep your fat-burning engines revving.

The Hormone Boost workout also has a significant effect on your T3 boost to support your weight loss. Because who feels like exercising when they're tired? I know it's a challenge for me when I feel sluggish. And that's how T3 helps—it increases your energy as it stimulates the metabolism of *every cell* in your body. This energy boost not only makes you feel like exercising, it also improves your performance while doing it! And the best news of all is that this sensation is nothing like a caffeine stimulant: T3 boosts your metabolic rate without side effects such as jitters. It simply energizes

According to study results from an overview of 1,164 individuals (with an average age of 34 years) published in the May 2015 edition of the journal *Clinical Chemistry*, turmeric just might be your secret weapon when it comes to thyroid health—especially in those with goiter. In 185 goiter subjects where TSH was measured, 92 had normal thyroid function, 91 had hyperthyroidism, and one subject each had hypothyroidism and subclinical hyperthyroidism. Goiter was significantly more common among females, unmarried individuals and individuals who drank tube-well (subterranean) water. Goiter was less common among those who consumed daily milk, daily ghee, spices, chilies and turmeric. Regular use of turmeric may be the key to reducing the risk of goiter. And let's be honest—incorporating spices like turmeric and green chilies into your diet makes for tasty meals too!

you, which means you don't experience the crash that comes from over-stimulation with stimulants.

Insulin Metabolism Boost

The evidence from a June 2015 study published in *Medical Science Monitor* is clear: The better your thyroid hormone status (and the lower your TSH), the better your insulin metabolism, which ultimately means fewer cravings and less belly fat. Since insulin is the only hormone that is always telling the body to store energy as fat, and is one of the most potent appetite-stimulating hormones, we never want to have too much insulin. So whether you have a diagnosed thyroid condition or not, the thyroid boost that you will experience from following the Hormone Boost gives you an advantage for fat loss in more ways than one.

Tips for a Thyroid Boost

Like so many other hormones, thyroid hormones must be present in the appropriate balance in order to ensure optimal health. As we've seen, these powerful communicators regulate our metabolism and organ function and directly affect heart rate, cholesterol levels, body weight, energy, muscle contraction and relaxation, skin and hair texture, bowel function, fertility, menstrual regularity, memory, mood and other body processes. The great news is that it's easy to stimulate your thyroid, and I'm going to tell you how.

Foods and Habits for Increased Thyroid Hormone

- **Sleep:** Aim for 7.5 to 9 hours of sleep. Not getting enough sleep decreases thyroid hormone, most likely because of the increased levels of cortisol associated with this state. Consecutive hours, rather than napping during the day, is best for stress-hormone balance and optimizing thyroid hormones.
- **Exercise:** The right amount of regular exercise increases thyroid hormone and prevents bouts of overexercising, which has been proven to increase cortisol and drop thyroid hormone for up to 24 hours (following a long, intense session). I have laid out the right amount of exercise for you in Chapter 12.
- **Avoid stress:** In addition to the meal and exercise plans included in this book, the Hormone Boost's simple steps in Chapter 8 will help you manage your stress levels. Remember: high levels of stress hormone (cortisol) block the activity of thyroid hormones and increase the risk of suboptimal thyroid function.
- **Get proper nutrition:** The Hormone Boost nutrition plan provides the right amounts of foods at the right times and in the right combinations to give your thyroid a boost. Skipping meals, severely restricting calories and denying yourself a "cheat meal" once a week can end up reducing the T3 that your body needs. Following the plan laid out in Part Three will ensure that you avoid these pitfalls and stay on track for optimum thyroid health. One way of doing this is to consume foods that contain the necessary nutrients to produce thyroid hormone, including:
  > **Tyrosine:** almonds, avocados, bananas, dairy products, pumpkin seeds and sesame seeds.

> **Iodine:** fish (cod, sea bass and haddock), shellfish and sea vegetables such as seaweed and kelp. Kelp is the richest source of iodine.

> **Selenium:** brewer's yeast, wheat germ, whole grains (barley, whole wheat, oats and brown rice), seeds, nuts (especially Brazil nuts), shellfish and some vegetables (garlic, onions, mushrooms, broccoli, tomatoes and radishes).

Supplement Options for a Thyroid Boost

In many cases, nutrients and herbs are required to increase the production and activity of thyroid hormone. These supplements can be taken safely with medications used to treat hypothyroidism (like Synthroid and Eltroxin). Clear Metabolism, which contains a combination of many of the individual ingredients listed below, is my favorite choice for a thyroid hormone boost.

- **Clear Metabolism – Thyroid Support Formula:** Wake up your metabolism with this fantastic formula that supports thyroid hormone production and activity. I have mixed the best thyroid-supporting ingredients together into one source, including iodine, potassium, L-tyrosine, ashwagandha, rosemary, forskohlin and gugulipids. Take 2 capsules daily upon rising, before breakfast (they can be taken at the same time as a thyroid medication).

- **Ashwagandha:** This supplement may increase both T4 and its more potent counterpart, T3. Both ashwagandha and gugulipids appear to boost thyroid function without influencing the release of the pituitary hormone TSH, indicating that these herbs work directly on the thyroid gland and other body tissues. Good news, since thyroid problems most often occur within the thyroid gland itself or in the conversion of T4 into T3 in tissues outside the thyroid gland. Take 750 to 1,000 mg twice daily. Ashwagandha is my favorite choice for supporting the thyroid when stress is also a concern.

- **Forskohlin:** Extracted from a plant called *Coleus forskohlii,* forskohlin may increase the release of thyroid hormone by stimulating a substance called cAMP. cAMP is comparable in strength to TSH, which prompts the thyroid to produce more thyroid hormone. Take 250 mg two to three times a day. *Coleus* is one of the top supplement choices when both weight loss and thyroid support are the goals.

- **Gugulipids:** Gugulipids (*Commiphora mukul*) enhance the conversion of T4 to the more potent T3. Dosage is 500 mg three times a day. Gugulipids may also lower elevated cholesterol and aid weight loss, so choose this one if you are concerned about high cholesterol or weight loss in addition to sluggish thyroid function.

- **L-tyrosine:** The amino acid tyrosine is necessary for the production of thyroid hormone in the body. The recommended dose is 1,000 to 2,000 mg upon rising, before breakfast. *Do not take this supplement if you have high blood pressure.*

- **Selenium:** A daily dose of 200 to 300 mcg of selenium (selenomethionine) can be helpful for cases of autoimmune thyroid disease and to support production of the active thyroid hormone T3.

- **BioThy (Biomed):** This mineral, amino acid and protein formula has been clinically identified as effective in cases of thyroid dysfunction (including hypothyroidism). It contains a nice blend of ingredients to boost thyroid hormones, including L-tyrosine (200 mg), iodine (kelp) (100 mcg), selenium (selenomethionine) (100 mcg), zinc (citrate) (10 mg) and animal thyroid protein hydrolysate and powder (bovine and porcine). Take 1 to 4 capsules daily upon rising. Testing your thyroid hormones after four weeks of using this product can be helpful to determine the right dose for you.

As the title of this chapter cheekily suggests, the thyroid hormone really *is* your metabolic master. It is a vital link in your system, and it's *hugely* important to understand its impact on your body. The suggestions above will help regulate the thyroid so that your whole system is healthy and working to its best capacity. But what about those times when we want to kick things up a notch? That's where adrenaline comes in.

A HORMONE BOOST REAL-LIFE SUCCESS STORY

THE CLIENT: Sharon S.

DETAILS: Female, 57

BODY COMPOSITION RESULTS (FROM SCALE AND BODY FAT/ MUSCLE MASS VIA BIO-IMPEDANCE TESTING)

MEASUREMENT	BEFORE	AFTER	TOTAL LOSS/GAIN
Weight (lb.)	143	128	(–) 15
Lean Body Mass (lb.)	98.5	96.5	(–) 2
Fat Mass (lb.)	44.5	31.5	(–) 13
Basal Metabolic Rate (calories/day)	1,395 calories	1,325 calories	(–) 70

Sharon was referred by James A., one of my favorite, most dynamic and incredibly talented patients—who is also an incredible success story of thyroid cancer survival. When Sharon arrived at my office in June 2015, she was experiencing pain in her arms, legs, hips, feet and neck. She also was taking medications for acid reflux and had been experiencing heartburn for over 20 years. She reported feeling stressed out, burned out and tired.

After just one month on the program, she lost 10 pounds, her pain had greatly diminished, her focus had improved and her heartburn had completely cleared! After five months of the Hormone Boost plan, her sleep was completely restored, she described her energy as "remarkable" and she attained her goal weight—all while maintaining her strength!

CHAPTER 2

FAT-LOSS HORMONE #2:
ACCELERATE WITH ADRENALINE

*I can't change the direction of the wind, but I can adjust
my sails to always reach my destination.*

JAMES DEAN, actor

Have you ever been startled or surprised? Most of us have, at some point or another. Just think about how your body responds: your pulse quickens, your muscles tense, your pupils dilate, your airways expand and your blood pressure spikes. These innate reactions are known as the fight-or-flight response, and they are designed to prepare you to protect yourself or run away. And all of them demonstrate what happens when adrenaline (also known as epinephrine) is at work.

Adrenaline Basics

The adrenal glands are two small glands that rest on top of the kidneys. They produce the stress hormones adrenaline and cortisol. When we're stressed—whether by information taken in and processed by our five senses or in relation to our thoughts—the body reacts by mounting a stress response through the stimulation of our sympathetic nervous system. So let's say your boss yells at you. What exactly happens, from a hormonal perspective?

- Your hypothalamus signals your pituitary gland to release

adrenocorticotropic hormone (ACTH).

- The ACTH, in turn, will stimulate the adrenal medulla to secrete adrenaline, and the adrenal cortex to secrete cortisol, among other hormones.
- Your cortisol level will increase and convert more stored glycogen than usual into blood sugar for energy. (Energy is also increased by the release of adrenaline from the adrenals.)
- Your heart rate will increase (from the adrenaline).
- You will tend to sweat more (from the cortisol).
- Your muscle tension will increase (from cortisol and adrenaline).
- Your digestion will slow down as blood is diverted to more important tissues.

Along with adrenaline, noradrenaline (NA, or norepinephrine) is released by nerve cells and the adrenal glands. NA also stimulates energy-expending fight-or-flight responses. Although it's typically not produced in as high a quantity as adrenaline, noradrenaline has very similar effects on body physiology, including increasing the heart rate, raising blood sugar and increasing tension in the skeletal muscles. It also stimulates the brain and helps us to think quickly when we are in tricky situations.

Here's the problem, though: Constantly overproducing adrenaline and cortisol can eventually lead to that all-too-familiar "burned out" feeling, also known as adrenal gland fatigue. The result is chronic exhaustion, lack of stamina for exercise, more allergy symptoms, lack of concentration, sleep disruption, blood sugar imbalance, weight gain, depression, increased cravings and weakened immunity.

How Adrenaline Works for You

So, too much adrenaline is a bad thing. But adrenaline in the right amounts at the right times can certainly offer real metabolic and hormonal benefits.

Fat-Loss Friend

When present in the right amounts, adrenaline is very useful in supporting fat loss. It causes the body to free up stored fats and sugars (a.k.a. glycogen), providing a burst of energy while sparing metabolically-active muscle protein. In today's day and age, when we don't often find ourselves having to escape from or face life-threatening danger, this energy burst can still be useful. Consider, for example, that having a cup of coffee before your workout may offer an extra fat-burning boost simply because caffeine sparks adrenaline production.

Blood Sugar Balancer

The complete digestion and absorption of a meal can take several hours, depending upon its size and composition. This means the carbs that end up as sugar (or glucose) in our bloodstream after a meal may also be available for several hours—and that's a good thing for our energy needs. But once the body's cells work through that glucose and no new sources are provided (like between meals or when fasting overnight), a new blood glucose scenario begins to take shape. When this happens, the pancreas releases the hormone glucagon. At the same time, adrenaline and cortisol promote efforts to help maintain blood glucose levels.

In skeletal muscle, slightly elevated adrenaline promotes the breakdown of glycogen to glucose. Unlike the glucose produced from the breakdown of liver glycogen, however, this glucose is not released into the blood. Rather, it remains in the muscle to become a supportive energy source for those muscle cells, while fat becomes the primary energy source for the rest of the body. This is great news for those of us working toward fat loss.

The hormone picture that develops during exercise is similar to the one that happens during a fasting period—with a few key differences. Adrenaline is released from our adrenal glands as a direct effect of exercise, depending on the type and intensity. In most cases, the greater your exercise intensity, the greater your adrenaline release. Both sprinting and circuit training, for instance, tend to stimulate adrenaline release. In turn, this adrenaline stimulates the breakdown of muscle-cell glycogen, making glucose available for those same cells (which are hard at work). Adrenaline also promotes the breakdown of glycogen to glucose in the liver, some of which will also circulate to working muscle.

Immune Booster

I know you've heard it a thousand times: Stress is bad for you. And it's certainly true that chronic stress, lasting weeks and months, has deleterious effects, including, notably, suppression of the immune response. But it turns out that short-term stress—the fight-or-flight response—actually stimulates immune activity. A 2014 study spearheaded by a Stanford University School of Medicine scientist has tracked the response of key immune cells in response to short-term stress. This research explored how hormones triggered by such stress enhance immune reactions. The study, conducted in rats, adds weight to evidence that immune responsiveness is *intensified*, rather than suppressed, as many believe, by the fight-or-flight response.

The study's findings provide an overview of how stress hormones affect the main cell types of the immune system. They also offer the prospect of someday being able to manipulate stress-hormone levels to improve patients' recovery from surgery, wounds or vaccine responses.

Our immune system is controlled by, among other things, the autonomic nervous system, which is involved in the fight-or-flight response that used to be thought of as involuntary. Experiments from intensive-care researcher Dr. Matthijs Kox and professor of experimental intensive care medicine Peter Pickkers, however, have now demonstrated that it is possible to purposely activate this system. With the help of breathing exercises, meditation and (interestingly) repeated exposure to cold, you can kick the autonomic nervous system into gear and inhibit an overactive immune system response. A well-functioning immune system protects our body from pathogens, but sometimes the immune response is too pronounced or persistent, and this can lead to the development of autoimmune diseases such as rheumatoid arthritis.

Mood Improver

According to a 2014 study published in *CNS & Neurological Disorders – Drug Targets*, depression can have an even greater influence on physical health than diabetes or arthritis. While treatment of depression normally involves antidepressants and psychotherapy, an international team of researchers found that sport and physical activity can produce almost as many beneficial changes as the traditionally-used medications.

We now know that sport and physical activity have a positive impact on the brain's serotonin activity, which brings about various changes that are otherwise achieved only through the use of drugs. Amazingly, a great workout or intense game strengthens adrenaline activity and ensures the release of various factors for nerve growth—factors that also promote cell growth in the brain and prevent cell death in the hippocampus caused by depression. Sport and physical activity also lead to reduced cortisol activity and ultimately cause an effect similar to that of mood-enhancing drugs—without the side effects!

Tips for an Adrenaline Boost

Accelerate your fat loss with the following simple tips to boost adrenaline.

Foods and Habits

- **Prioritize proper nutrition:** To increase your adrenaline hormone, incorporate coffee, tea, green tea, citrus fruits, bananas, chocolate, cocoa and vanilla into your diet.

- **Exercise:** Interval training, such as sprinting, boosts adrenaline. In a study published in *Medicine & Science in Sports & Exercise* (2005), researchers found that a group of test subjects who worked out continuously, with no rest between exercises (i.e., circuit training), had greater increases in growth hormone, noradrenaline and adrenaline during their workouts. They also netted greater muscle gains after 12 weeks than those who were instructed to rest between exercises.
- **Turn up the music:** Listening to exciting music can increase the release of adrenaline into your bloodstream, giving you yet another reason to add tunes to your workout (or hit a dance club)!

Supplement Options

- **Clear Vive:** Pop one capsule of this powerful product and I promise you will feel a boost in your energy and focus in about 20 to 30 minutes. It is the strongest energy supplement I have in my Clear Medicine line. Taken before a workout, it's an incredible way to increase fat-burning efforts, thanks to the boost of adrenaline and adiponectin it offers. The main ingredients that lead to these benefits are essential oils (EPA, DHA and GLA), green tea, theanine and green coffee bean extract. Do not take this product after 3 p.m., as it will keep you awake.
- **Vitamins B$_5$ and B$_6$:** These important B vitamins play an integral role in cell metabolism. Improving your metabolic pathways boosts your energy levels and is a great way to reduce fatigue. B$_5$ helps to produce coenzyme A, which contributes to cellular respiration and the breakdown of fats, proteins and carbohydrates. B$_6$ acts in several of the pathways that are used to create adrenal hormones. Take a B complex like Thorne Research B-Complex #6 or Clear B Boost—one capsule at breakfast or lunch.

- **Clear C:** This powerful antioxidant vitamin is directly involved in the production of hormones in your adrenals. So, besides the other health benefits it provides (boosting your immune system, protecting from free radicals), vitamin C is also an essential building block for adrenal gland recovery. You can start with 1,000 mg daily and then gradually increase your dose over time. Buffered or liposomal vitamin C is generally the best form, and it should be in combination with bioflavonoids, just as it often is in nature. Clear C contains a mixture of vitamin C and black pepper, to enhance vitamin absorption.

- **Synephrine (*Citrus aurantium*):** Synephrine is an alkaloid that occurs naturally in very small amounts in humans and plants, but it is also made synthetically for use in some adrenergic drugs. The biggest supplier of supplemented synephrine in the world is the tree *Citrus aurantium*, which is native to southeast Asia. A June 2015 study in the *International Journal of Food Sciences and Nutrition* included overweight men who received 900 mg of a citrus-based polyphenol extract, Sinetrol-XPur, daily for 12 weeks. Body composition, anthropometric and blood parameters were assessed before and after the intervention period. The study showed that taking 450 mg twice daily (at breakfast and lunch) for 12 weeks resulted in a 5.8-pound average weight loss and a 6.6 percent reduction in body fat, while placebo subjects experienced no significant weight or body-fat loss. The extract group also lost an average of two inches off their waist and hip circumference.

- **Clear Energy:** This formula contains two amino acid building blocks of adrenaline, L-tyrosine and DL-phenylalanine. L-tyrosine supplements appear to be protective for acute stressors (which tend to deplete adrenaline) and may prevent stress-induced memory deficits. I recommend a dose of three

Clear Energy capsules or 500 to 1,500 mg of L-tyrosine per day upon rising.

Adrenaline is a provocateur; it provokes you into fight-or-flight responses, thus accelerating your ability to burn fat. But as we've seen, it doesn't just work physically. It also provokes your brain, stimulating it to work harder. And because it mobilizes your body's resources in the short term, it also stimulates immune system activity. So now that you've got all the info you need to "rev up," let's get our androgenic motors running!

A HORMONE BOOST REAL-LIFE SUCCESS STORY

THE CLIENT: Marilyn K.

DETAILS: Female, 42

BODY COMPOSITION RESULTS (FROM SCALE AND BODY FAT/ MUSCLE MASS VIA BIO-IMPEDANCE TESTING)

MEASUREMENT	BEFORE	AFTER	TOTAL LOSS/GAIN
Weight (lb.)	139.2	129	(-) 10.2
Lean Body Mass (lb.)	90.9	91.2	(+) 0.3
Fat Mass (lb.)	48.3	41.0	(-) 7.3
Basal Metabolic Rate (calories/day)	1,285 calories	1,289 calories	(+) 4

Marilyn is a sharp travel agent with a smile that never disappears. We love seeing her at Clear Medicine whenever she pops in! Over the course of six weeks, this lovely lady lost 10 pounds of fat and gained 1.4 pounds of muscle. Her insomnia cleared up, her energy improved and her migraines became less frequent.

CHAPTER 3

FAT-LOSS HORMONE #3:
THE ANDROGENIC HORMONES
DHEA AND TESTOSTERONE

*All the adversity I've had in my life, all my troubles and obstacles,
have strengthened me . . . You may not realize it when it happens,
but a kick in the teeth may be the best thing in the world for you.*

WALT DISNEY

Androgens are a group of hormones that include testosterone, DHEA and androsterone. Although often referred to as the male hormones, androgens are present in different amounts in men and women. Males, however, naturally make greater bodily amounts than women, producing them primarily in the testes; women generate a small amount in the ovaries.

DHEA Basics

Produced by the adrenal glands, dehydroepiandrosterone (DHEA) is a precursor to the sex hormones estrogen and testosterone, and one of the most abundant hormones in our bodies. This hormone with the very long name has an equally long list of benefits. It's known to support healthy immunity (particularly for the prevention of autoimmune imbalances), aid tissue repair, improve sleep and counteract the negative effects of cortisol. It influences our ability to lose fat and gain muscle. And it boosts libido and helps us feel motivated, youthful and energetic. For all of these reasons and more, DHEA is often touted as the anti-aging hormone. DHEA naturally declines with age, stress and illness, and it is often taken in supplements.

How DHEA Works for You

Keeping your DHEA in the optimal range offers a host of benefits for your heart, brain, bones and body composition. You can measure your DHEA levels in blood or saliva. Optimal levels should be above 225 mcg/dL or, more specifically, 300 to 400 mcg/dL for men and 225 to 350 mcg/dL for women. Now let's dive a little deeper into the benefits of boosting your DHEA into the optimal range.

Androgen Excess

Normally our bodies keep androgens perfectly balanced with the female hormones (estrogen and progesterone), but sometimes a woman's body can produce too much, resulting in a situation known as androgen excess. Androgen excess is seen primarily in women during the reproductive years, from early adolescence to the start of menopause. Many women with androgen excess have a condition known as polycystic ovary syndrome (PCOS)—a condition I am all too familiar with (I received my diagnosis in 1999).

Bone Builder

A 2009 study from Saint Louis University found that taking DHEA hormone supplements, in conjunction with calcium and vitamin D, could lower the risk of spine fractures in older women by 30 to 50 percent. Earlier studies had not shown such promising results, but it appears that calcium and vitamin D deficiencies, which are present in half of older adults, may have prevented DHEA from improving bone density in those cases. Combining all three supplements rather than relying on their individual effects seems to do more.

Another group of researchers, however, wanted to establish whether DHEA replacement therapy might be useful in the treatment of steroid-induced osteoporosis in women. In June 2012, *Advances in Medical Sciences* published the results of a study that had recruited 19 women, aged 50 to 78, to be treated for at least three years with average daily doses of more than 7.5 mg of prednisone. For the first year of the study, the patients were given calcium, vitamin D_3 and thiazide diuretics. For the second year, the patients received a dose of orally micronized DHEA (25 to 50 mg daily). Serum concentrations of DHEA-S, androstenedione, testosterone, estradiol, growth hormone (IGF-1) and osteocalcin (all of which contribute to stronger, healthier bones) were assessed before the study, after 12 months of calcium and vitamin D_3 therapy, and then after six weeks and six months of DHEA therapy. Bone mineral density in the lumbar spine and femoral neck was also measured before the treatment, after one year on calcium and vitamin D_3, and after six and 12 months of DHEA replacement therapy.

In all participants, DHEA significantly increased serum DHEA-S, androstenedione and testosterone concentrations. As early as six weeks after DHEA treatment began, the study reported a significant elevation of serum growth hormone and osteocalcin concentrations. Similarly, a significant increase of bone mineral density in the lumbar spine and femoral neck was observed after six and twelve months of DHEA treatment. Because osteoporosis is a common risk associated with the use of corticosteroid medications, a treatment protocol that includes calcium, vitamin D_3 and DHEA to reduce this risk makes good sense for strong bones.

Muscle Protector

Sarcopenia is a condition characterized by progressive and generalized loss of muscle mass and strength, and it carries the risk of adverse outcomes such as physical disability, poor quality of life and even death. This condition is linked to a number of causes, including declining levels of DHEA and testosterone. There is good news, however: A study published in the January 2013 issue of *Current*

Opinion in Clinical Nutrition and Metabolic Care found that boosting DHEA and, more important, testosterone, is associated with increased muscle mass.

Researchers continue to explore the muscle-related benefits of DHEA. One recent study reveals how DHEA protects muscle. During five days of successive exercise training, 16 young male participants (19 to 21 years old) received either a placebo or a DHEA supplement (100 mg daily). The results of this research, which appeared in the *European Journal of Applied Physiology* (January 2013), showed that training increased circulating creatine kinase (CK) levels, a marker in the blood of muscle damage, by approximately ninefold in the placebo group. In the DHEA-supplemented group, only a threefold increase was observed. This suggests that DHEA may play a role in protecting skeletal muscles from exercise-induced damage.

Fertility Booster

Scientists have found a statistical connection between the vitamin supplement DHEA, used to counter the effects of aging, and successful pregnancy rates in women undergoing treatment for infertility. In the first controlled study (reported from Tel Aviv University in July 2010) on the effects of the supplement, researchers found that women being treated for infertility who also received DHEA supplements were three times more likely to conceive than women being treated without the additional hormone.

Tips to Boost DHEA

DHEA offers a dose of anti-aging, anti-stress, fertility, immune-bolstering and bone-building benefits. Here's how to get yours:

Foods and Habits

- **Meditate:** According to Deepak Chopra, MD, meditation is proven to increase the production of DHEA and boost serotonin, our feel-good hormone. I highly recommend guided meditations (check on YouTube) or activities that involve repetitive motion, which can also be meditative, like walking or cycling.

- **Exercise (specifically weight training):** Unlike cardiovascular exercise, strength training increases DHEA. This is just one reason why I've included a fantastic weekly training program for you in Part Three.
- **Have sex—regularly:** Orgasms spark an anti-aging surge of DHEA. So consider this medical advice: Having at least two orgasms a week can slow the aging process and indirectly support fat loss, while also offering some protection from the adverse effects of cortisol.
- **Sleep well and enough:** Sleeping regenerates the adrenal glands, which produce DHEA, and helps to reduce cortisol, especially when you get to sleep before 10 p.m. (The adrenal glands are truly resting between the hours of 10 p.m. and 2 a.m.)
- **Manage stress:** With advancing age and higher stress, cortisol increases and DHEA decreases. So remember this: Anything that cuts cortisol helps DHEA do its protective and regenerative work. Anything we do, think, say or feel can either stress us or calm us—so think happy thoughts and live for sensory bliss.

Supplement Options

I support the use of DHEA supplements, but *only* in low doses, and *only* when a true deficiency has been definitively diagnosed via blood or saliva testing. Taking too much DHEA can trigger an unwelcome increase in testosterone and estrogen, which leads to increased cancer risk, hair loss, anger, aggression and acne in both men and women. Women may also experience effects such as a deeper voice, hair loss and abnormal growth of facial hair. So, if you've got the deficiency diagnosis in hand, consider the following options.

- **Clear Balance – Stress Support Formula:** The main ingredient of this formula is Relora, which has been shown in studies to significantly reduce cortisol and raise DHEA within only two weeks of use (without the risk of causing excessive DHEA). Relora can be used to prevent the health conditions associated with stress, including poor immunity, high blood pressure, insomnia or sleep disruption, loss of vitality and weight gain, especially in relation to metabolic syndrome. Take two 250 mg capsules at bedtime and one upon rising, away from food. In my experience, the most effective Relora formula should contain a mixture of B vitamins and folic acid, just as the Clear Balance – Stress Support Formula does.
- **DHEA:** You can purchase DHEA supplements over the counter in the United States, but its sale is restricted in Canada. DHEA should be taken only under supervision by a licensed health-care provider. I prefer low dosages of 5 to 25 mg twice daily with meals. You should test your DHEA levels after four to six weeks of using the supplement to avoid taking excessive amounts, which can be harmful.
- **7-keto-DHEA:** Unlike straight DHEA, 7-keto-DHEA does not convert to estrogen or testosterone, making it a good choice for younger people, who in most cases would not benefit from increased amounts of these hormones. 7-keto has documented metabolism-enhancing effects, promotes fat loss, protects us from the harmful effects of excess cortisol and appears to prevent the decrease in metabolism known to occur when we're dieting. Take 25 to 100 mg twice a day. The higher dosage has been proven effective for weight loss in clinical trials, according to a report in *Current Therapeutic Research* (2000).

- **Royal jelly:** I always thought that royal jelly (a secretion created by worker honeybees) seemed like a gimmicky supplement, but a 2012 study suggests that it just might have some real hormone-boosting benefits. Published in *Nutrition Journal's* September 2012 edition, this study included a total of 61 healthy volunteers aged 42 to 83, who were randomly divided into a royal jelly group and a control group. For a period of six months, 3,000 mg of royal jelly or a placebo in 100 ml of liquid was ingested daily by the respective groups. The results showed that six months of ingesting royal jelly improved the production of red blood cells, glucose tolerance and mental health. Researchers concluded that increased testosterone and DHEA production led to these favorable results.

Given the benefits associated with DHEA—anti-aging, fertility, bone health, muscle strength—a low-dose supplement after a deficiency diagnosis seems like a no-brainer.

Testosterone Basics

Testosterone is produced by the ovaries in women, the testes in men and the adrenal glands in both sexes. While you are under stress your body will tend to make more stress hormone (cortisol) than testosterone. Considering low testosterone, in both sexes, has been linked to depression, obesity, osteoporosis, heart disease and even death (in men), it's certainly a boost to strive for. Researchers have found that men with low testosterone are more likely to develop a potbelly and other body fat, yet replacing testosterone may prompt the loss of body fat. Signs of low testosterone such as loss of muscle tissue; depression; and decreased strength, stamina, drive and motivation, suggest a need for a testosterone top-up and make having it tested good medical sense. If you have your testosterone levels assessed, be sure to request blood tests for both free and total testosterone.

How Testosterone Works for You

Loss of testosterone with aging can lead to andropause, often referred to as male menopause. This condition is estimated to affect about 30 percent of aging men, although actual numbers may be much higher, because the widely varying symptoms make definitive diagnosis difficult. Common symptoms include fatigue, depression, loss of muscle mass, forgetfulness, low libido and more. I should add that these effects can arise in both in men and women, even with dieting and exercise, when a marked deficiency of testosterone exists. On the other hand, a boost of testosterone, classically thought of as the driver of strength and vigor, offers a myriad of other benefits too, as our mood, bones, waist size and memory are all impacted by this powerful hormone.

Does Testosterone Boost a Man's Honesty?

A 2012 study from the University of Bonn demonstrated that testosterone—the sex hormone associated with upright posture and aggression—also, surprisingly, fosters social behavior. Researchers found that participants in the study who had received testosterone lied less frequently during play situations than individuals who had received only a placebo.

Mood Enhancer

Testosterone appears to have antidepressant properties, and now scientists have discovered that a specific pathway in the hippocampus—a brain region involved in memory formation and the regulation of stress responses—may play a major role in mediating testosterone's effects, according to a report in *Biological Psychiatry* (2012).

Women are twice as likely as men to suffer from an affective disorder like depression. Men with hypogonadism, a condition where the body produces no or low testosterone, also suffer increased levels of depression and anxiety. In these patients, testosterone replacement therapy has been shown to effectively improve mood.

Red wine could give athletes a boost by increasing the amount of performance-enhancing testosterone in their bodies, according to researchers from London's Kingston University, whose study results were reported in *Nutrition Journal* (2012).

A team led by Professor Declan Naughton, from the university's School of Life Sciences, found that red wine may reduce the amount of testosterone excreted by the body, which could distort the findings of drug tests taken from urine samples. Since testosterone can increase muscle mass, boost stamina and speed up recovery, athletes are prohibited from taking it, or a synthetic version of it, to try to gain a competitive edge.

The team found that a compound in red wine, known as quercetin, partially blocked the action of an enzyme that looks for testosterone and then sends a message to the kidneys to excrete it. It's tough to tell how much red wine would be needed to achieve this result, as the effect on an individual would vary by weight, fitness level, current health status and dietary habits. The same results were, however, noted for quercetin in supplement form, if ever you are in need of anti-doping tricks. (I kid!)

Although it may seem as if we know a great deal about depression, it is vitally important to fully characterize how and where in the brain these effects are occurring, so scientists can better target the development of future antidepressant therapies. Studies like this suggest that we need to move beyond simply focusing on boosting serotonin with SSRI medications to improve mood and treat depression. Fully exploring a multi-faceted hormone-health approach—like the Hormone Boost—could have significant results.

Weight-Loss (and Waist-Size) Aid

A study examining testosterone-deficient men revealed that they experienced major weight loss during (and up to five years after) testosterone replacement therapy. These results, presented at the June 2012 Endocrine Society's 94th annual meeting in Houston, note that participants received subcutaneous testosterone by injection for 18 weeks. The men lost weight continuously during treatment and, more than five years after the treatment stopped, they'd lost more than 35 pounds of body weight! Studies like this demonstrate the clear relationship between testosterone deficiency and obesity—particularly abdominal adipose tissue, which produces a number of substances that suppress testosterone production.

According to the data, the mean weight loss was 4.12 percent after one year, 7.47 percent after two years, 9.01 percent after three years, 11.26 percent after four years and 13.21 percent after five years. Although prior studies using testosterone therapy in testosterone-deficient men consistently showed changes in body composition, such as increased lean mass and decreased fat mass, the net effect on weight seemed unchanged. This study, however, had a longer follow-up by at least two years and used long-acting injections of testosterone. And this is exactly the reason why I want everyone who begins the Hormone Boost plan to get a testosterone boost over the long term—and at any age!

Even more favorable results on testosterone were presented at that same Endocrine Society meeting. Another study found that, in addition to testosterone increasing weight loss in testosterone-deficient men, weight loss can reduce the prevalence of low testosterone levels in overweight middle-aged men with prediabetes by almost 50 percent. Testosterone increases weight loss; weight loss increases testosterone—that's a win-win situation, and a definitive reason to get started on this plan.

Overweight men with low testosterone levels often try to lose weight through diet and exercise *before* turning to testosterone therapy to raise their hormone levels. This study advocates for a simultaneous approach. The reciprocal relationship among diet, exercise and testosterone reinforces the benefits of addressing these three areas together. (Remember, testosterone increases weight loss; weight loss increases testosterone; and exercise increases both!)

Whenever I do TV and speaking engagements, I wear red undies or a red bra. Why? For the same reason so many athletes choose to wear red when they compete (e.g., Tiger Woods famously chooses to wear a red shirt on the last day of major competitions). A study published in *Psychological Science* (May 2013) suggests that the color may be linked to our testosterone levels.

Apparently, males who chose to wear red during a competitive task had higher testosterone levels than males who chose blue. Choosing to wear red may unconsciously signal something about our competitive nature, and it may well be something that affects how our opponents respond. Funnily enough, choosing red did not seem to have an impact on personal performance in the study's competitive task. Instead, researchers believe that direct competition, in which opponents can be seen wearing red or appearing red, may be necessary for the red advantage to occur. Along these lines, previous research has shown that wearing red can be advantageous through its influence on opponents' perceptions, leading them to view red competitors as being "high quality."

Now you know: For your next big "game" (whether it's a personal or a professional moment where you want to shine), go for red—on top or underneath—even if only for a boost in mental confidence.

Strength Builder

Hulk out: A 2011 study published in the *Journal of Clinical Endocrinology & Metabolism* found that higher levels of testosterone were associated with reduced loss of lean muscle mass in older men, especially in those who were losing weight. In these men, aged 65 and older, higher testosterone levels were also associated with greater retention of lower body strength.

Loss of muscle mass and strength contributes to frailty and is associated with falls, mobility limitations and fractures. Men lose more muscle mass and strength than women as they age (simply because they start off with more), suggesting that sex steroids, and testosterone in particular, may contribute to body composition and physical function changes.

The men in this study who had higher testosterone levels lost less muscle mass, especially in their arms and legs, than study participants who had lower testosterone levels. Men who had higher testosterone levels before they lost weight also lost less leg function and could stand up more easily from a chair than men who had lower testosterone levels before they lost weight.

Tips for a Testosterone Boost

Testosterone enhances libido, bone density, muscle mass, strength, motivation, memory, fat burning and skin tone. In men, it influences sperm production, causes growth of the prostate gland and is especially important for maintaining motivation and mood.

As with so many other hormones, testosterone levels tend to taper off with aging, obesity and stress. Exposure to pesticides and toxins also negatively impacts the production of testosterone in the testes. Today, men are experiencing testosterone decline much earlier in life, and overall levels appear to be dropping. All the more reason to give this important hormone a boost.

Foods and Habits

- **Sleep:** The right amount of sleep impacts testosterone levels, so try to get the shut-eye your body needs. Sleep-deprived men and women have lower testosterone levels, and individuals with sleep apnea are also known to have testosterone deficiencies.
- **Exercise:** Both aerobic and strength training boost testosterone.
- **Have sex:** Women appear to get a testosterone boost simply from cuddling, while men seem to require actual sex.
- **Walk in the sun:** Go outside! Exposure to morning sunlight is a fantastically simple way for both men and women to boost testosterone levels.

- **Consume protein and carbohydrates:** Consuming adequate protein and sufficient fat while avoiding excessive carbohydrate restriction is critical to maintaining testosterone levels. Complete carb restriction reduces testosterone and increases cortisol—which only serves to further reduce testosterone. This is *not* what we want! Insulin is released in response to carbohydrates in our diet. Insulin may also help prevent further breakdown of muscle tissue after a workout, through its enhancing action on testosterone. This hormone is vital to the growth and maintenance of muscle tissue. In the right amount, insulin prevents the body from breaking down proteins, such as those found in muscle tissue, for energy during times of stress. Without insulin, your cells would not have access to enough amino acids, glucose and fatty acids to survive, let alone grow, heal and repair. So eat your carbs (like those in fruits or in the beta-berry and natural beet sweetener extracts included in Clear Recovery – Sports and Energy Formula) and protein (such as Dream Protein) mixed together post-workout for a testosterone and muscle boost.
- **Play sports:** Taking part in any competitive physical activity provides a testosterone boost, especially for men. (Don't forget to wear red!)
- **Enjoy success:** In business, competitive activities and new adventures are found to enhance testosterone in men. Perhaps you have noticed this before, ladies, when your husband comes home with his chest puffed up from a competitive day at the office.

Supplement Options
- **Clear Libido Boost – Hormonal Balance Formula (formerly called Clear Testosterone):** Clear Libido Boost contains a nice blend of herbs to support the body during stress (a major killer of testosterone), and other herbs that help promote

optimal testosterone production and function. Take one to three capsules daily upon rising, away from food.

- **Bio-identical testosterone cream:** See your doctor, naturopath or compounding pharmacy.
- **Clear Detox – Hormonal Health:** Excess estrogen is often associated with a testosterone deficiency in men. My detox formulation can support higher testosterone levels, since it helps with the removal of harmful estrogen.
- *Tribulus terrestris:* Also known as puncture vine, *Tribulus* may boost testosterone by increasing the pituitary gland's secretion of luteinizing hormone (LH), the hormone that stimulates production of testosterone. Other studies suggest it boosts testosterone by increasing DHEA. Take 500 to 1,000 mg daily, away from food.
- **Arginine:** Arginine may improve testosterone (and blood flow; in fact, it's often referred to as "natural Viagra"). Take 3,000 mg daily, away from food, preferably at bedtime.
- **Zinc:** This mineral is needed to maintain testosterone levels in the blood. A zinc deficiency causes a decrease in the activity of LH. Zinc also appears to inhibit the conversion of testosterone to estrogen via the aromatase enzyme. Take 25 to 50 mg daily with food.

You get extra points if you can remember DHEA's *loooong* full name! Even if you can't, you are sure to remember its ability to support our immune system, repair tissue, facilitate sleep and counteract cortisol. It also helps us lose fat, gain muscle and boost libido. When combined with the boosting power of testosterone (which isn't just for men!), DHEA ensures that our bodies have denser bones, more muscle mass and less fat. We're stronger and more motivated, and our memory improves. Together, these two hormones invigorate us inside and out. You may find that you want that kind of invigoration to last—which is why we have to talk about growth hormone and acetylcholine.

A HORMONE BOOST REAL-LIFE SUCCESS STORY

THE CLIENT: MariaLisa D.

DETAILS: Female, 43

**BODY COMPOSITION RESULTS (FROM SCALE AND BODY FAT/
MUSCLE MASS VIA BIO-IMPEDANCE TESTING)**

MEASUREMENT	BEFORE	AFTER	TOTAL LOSS/GAIN
Weight (lb.)	130	121	(-) 9
Lean Body Mass (lb.)	98.1	101.4	(+) 3.3
Fat Mass (lb.)	31.9	19.6	(-) 12.3
Basal Metabolic Rate (calories/day)	1,388 calories	1,426 calories	(+) 38

Can you say *drop-dead gorgeous*? Because that's what comes to mind when I look at this perfect example of Hormone Boost success. MariaLisa is a dancer and a mother of three—and she is now also absolutely ripped!

She originally came to me with some anxiety, irritability, sugar cravings at 3 p.m. and 9 p.m., fatigue, bloating, cramping and weight gain. Check out her body transformation results! Her hard work within the Hormone Boost program has allowed her to gain 3.3 pounds of muscle and drop 12.3 pounds of fat. Her energy is excellent; she sleeps well; her mood is stable and balanced. She no longer experiences anxiety, bloating, PMS or irritability—and she's super chilled out. (I think she's pretty wise too.)

Love this lady! If I could put her on a postcard as the Hormone Boost's promise of results, it would be a marketing dream.

CHAPTER 4

FAT-LOSS HORMONE #4:
GROWTH HORMONE AND ACETYLCHOLINE
HORMONES OF STRENGTH AND REJUVENATION

*Success is going from failure to failure
without losing your enthusiasm.*

WINSTON CHURCHILL

Growth hormone (GH) affects just about every cell in the body. Not surprisingly, it also has a major effect on our feelings, actions and appearance. Because this regenerative hormone tends to decline with age, GH supplements are often promoted as a way to slow the effects of aging.

GH Basics

GH is released during deep sleep and while we exercise. It's essential for tissue repair, muscle building, bone density and healthy body composition. When we sleep in total darkness, melatonin is released, triggering a very slight but critical cool-down in the body. As our body temperature drops, GH is released and works its regenerative magic. If we sleep with the lights on or eat too close to bedtime, the natural cool-down process will not take place, putting us at risk for low levels of both melatonin and GH. We are also in

Only recently has adult GH deficiency been recognized as a serious health problem. Abdominal obesity in postmenopausal women has been linked to low GH secretion, elevated inflammatory markers and increased risk of cardiovascular disease. Test subjects in an April 2007 *Journal of Clinical Endocrinology & Metabolism* study received supplementary GH—and demonstrated improvement in inflammatory markers as a result. And researchers at Saint Louis University also found that obese people who received controlled doses of GH lost weight while maintaining the energy to exercise.

danger of losing the important effects of sleep on fat loss.

Once released into the bloodstream, GH has a very short life—only a half-hour or so. During that time, however, it makes its way speedily to the liver and many other cells in the body, inducing them to produce another hormone, called insulin-like growth factor 1 (IGF-1). Almost every cell in the body is affected by IGF-1, especially muscle, bone, liver, kidney, skin, lung and nerve cells. Commonly measured as a marker of GH production, IGF-1 is the substance truly responsible for most of the restorative benefits we typically attribute to GH.

How GH Works for You

GH replacement unequivocally benefits growth, body composition, cardiovascular risk factors and quality of life. Less commonly known benefits of this rejuvenating hormone include enhancements in learning and memory, brain power and performance.

Learning and Memory Aid

According to a June 2010 study published in the *Journal of Endocrinology*, treatment to increase GH has been associated with improvements in measures of memory and attention. But, while beneficial for both men and women, it turns out that GH has different effects depending on sex. According to a piece in the *Proceedings of the National Academy of Sciences* (March 2006), GH is produced within the hippocampus. Found deep inside your brain, the hippocampus is involved with memory and emotion.

More GH was produced in females than in males, and more in adults than in children. Interestingly, greater amounts of GH were also produced in response to estrogen, which may have implications for menopausal women using estrogen replacement therapy (which certainly seems like a good reason to use bio-identical hormone replacement) and for athletes taking GH and anabolic steroids to increase muscle mass.

We know from previous studies that hippocampal GH increases with learning (after all the research and learning I have done for this book, my GH levels must be awesome). The 2006 study, though, also shows that the levels of GH in the brain increased with stress, particularly in males, while the effect in females depended on how much estrogen they had at the time. So it seems that sex hormones like estrogen have a tremendous effect on the growth and architecture of the brain, and may explain some of the differences in how males and females learn.

Brain-Power Booster
According to a clinical trial published by *Archives of Neurology* (2012), IGF-1 has potent effects on brain function. The decrease in GH that occurs with advancing age likely plays a role in the pathogenesis of Alzheimer's disease. This study, involving 153 patients with mild cognitive impairments (MCI), lasted 20 weeks. Analysis after the 20-week mark showed a favorable effect of IGF-1 on cognition, which was comparable in both adults with MCI and healthy older adults. And that's good news: GH gives a brain boost!

Weekend Warrior Performance Enhancer
The benefits of GH are not solely for the elderly or obese. A study released in the *Annals of Internal Medicine* in 2010 found that GH also improved sprint capacity in healthy recreational athletes. During

the 8-week study, 96 recreationally trained athletes aged 18 to 40 (63 men and 33 women) were randomly assigned to receive either an inactive placebo or a GH injection. At the same time, half of the male participants were also randomly assigned to receive an additional injection of placebo or testosterone.

At the 8-week mark, researchers found that GH injections increased the athletes' ability to sprint on a bicycle, but it had no effect on overall fitness or the ability to pull a weight or jump. Interestingly, the effect on sprint capacity nearly doubled in the men who also received testosterone injections. In addition to improvements in sprint capacity, researchers found that GH significantly reduced fat mass among the athletes but did not seem to increase muscle mass. The elevated sprint capacity returned to normal six weeks after participants stopped receiving injections.

Different growth hormones respond to exercise differently. A study published in the *American Journal of Physiology – Endocrinology and Metabolism* (December 2006) found that GH was responsive to moderate and heavy exercise regimens with three to twelve repetitions of varying weights. Sounds like my good old Hormone Diet workout—which, in my experience, is still the best way for women to strength-train (the plan starts with light and moves to heavier weights by the third set). Having a heavy loading cycle or workout in resistance-training routines really is the secret to building muscle and bone. Because this style of training creates the greatest potentiation of GH levels in women, exercising any other way just won't reap the maximum rewards.

Men, on the other hand, rely to a greater extent on muscle-building testosterone. Since women rely on GH to increase muscle and bone strength, the more GH stimulated by a type of exercise, the better its outcome. But these are not the only benefits—GH also plays a role in fighting tissue breakdown, staving off stress fractures and improving metabolic function.

Keep in mind that an injection is not the only way to get a GH boost; all aspects of the Hormone Boost plan help foster this result—especially the workout, sleep rules and diet plan.

Tips to Boost GH

Given that GH affects just about every cell in the body, it's not surprising that it also has a major effect on our feelings, actions and appearance. We need to do what we can to make sure we're giving this important hormone a boost.

Foods and Habits

- **Sleep:** A no-brainer—get some! But you must follow my Hormone Boost rules outlined in Chapter 8.
- **Exercise:** Exercise is essential to the production of GH. The Hormone Boost workout in Chapter 12 outlines exactly what you need to stimulate GH.
- **Get the right nutrition:** Consume sufficient lean protein. Specific guidelines can be found in Chapter 10.
- **Avoid stress:** Because cortisol suppresses GH, it's important to manage your daily stresses. Yoga, meditation, hobbies, sex—whatever alleviates your stress and allows you to relax is worth your time and energy.
- **Try fasting:** There has been a lot of discussion recently about the benefits of fasting. And science backs this up: Cardiac researchers at the Intermountain Medical Center Heart Institute (May 2011) have demonstrated that routine periodic fasting is good for our health and our hearts. This discovery expands upon a 2007 Intermountain Healthcare study that revealed an association between fasting and a reduced risk of coronary heart disease, the leading cause of death among men and women in the United States. Fasting was also found to reduce other cardiac risk factors, such as triglycerides, weight and blood sugar levels. Apparently the hunger or

stress caused by fasting leads the body to release more cholesterol, which allows it to utilize fat as a source of fuel, instead
of glucose. Ultimately, then, this decreases the number of fat
cells in the body. GH protects lean muscle and metabolic balance, a response triggered and accelerated by fasting. During
the 24-hour fasting periods undertaken in the study, GH
increased an average of 1,300 percent in women and nearly
2,000 percent in men. However you feel about the "hanger"
or stress of fasting, these results suggest that you may want to
(gently and slowly) incorporate fasting into your lifestyle.

- **Laugh:** Interestingly enough, laughter boosts GH. That
means you have scientific motivation to watch the latest com-
edy! (You're welcome.)

Supplement Options

- **Clear Recovery:** Out of all my formulations, this might be
my favorite. Complete with three types of glutamine, creati-
nine, branched-chain amino acids, resveratrol, berry
extracts, minerals and loads of antioxidants, it aids recovery
after exercise and supports the production of GH. Take one
serving in water after exercise, or in the mid-afternoon if
you need an energy boost. If you are extremely athletic, you
can take two servings during or after weight-training sessions
or endurance exercise.

- **Specific amino acids:** The amino acid precursors to GH are
arginine, lysine, ornithine and glutamine. Supplements of
these amino acids taken together before bed or after exercise
may be useful to support GH production. Aim for the following dosages:
    > *L-arginine:* 2,000 to 3,000 mg per day
    > *L-glutamine:* 2,000 mg per day
    > *L-ornithine:* 2,000 to 6,000 mg per day
    > *L-lysine:* 1,200 mg per day

> *L-glycine:* 1,000 mg per day

> *L-tyrosine:* 1,000 mg per day

These amino acids are most effective when combined with vitamin B_3, vitamin B_6, vitamin C, calcium, zinc and potassium.

- **IGF² Growth Factor (ATP Labs):** I love this formula! Its alpha-GPC, L-tyrosine and acetyl-L-carnitine provide a nice boost of both acetylcholine and GH. A precursor of the neurotransmitter acetylcholine, alpha-GPC is used to treat Alzheimer's disease, loss of cognitive function and memory loss. Unlike phosphatidylcholines (see page 75), alpha-GPC easily crosses the blood–brain barrier to improve our brain cell health. Among athletes, alpha-GPC increases endurance and performance. It can also boost GH production by stimulating the regeneration of pituitary gland functions. Tyrosine is a non-essential amino acid that plays a role in the synthesis of catecholamines: epinephrine, norepinephrine, dopamine and DOPA. It is also a precursor of melanin (the pigment that colors the skin, hair and irises) and thyroid hormones. Acetyl-L-carnitine, an acetylated form of L-carnitine, is a natural by-product of the lysine amino acid. Acetyl-L-carnitine easily passes through the blood–brain barrier and is an antioxidant helpful in maintaining good health. An amino acid known for its role in muscle growth and development, fat loss, increased energy and improved resistance to muscle fatigue, it also reduces the sensation of hunger. So it can play a critical metabolic role in stimulating your weight loss by contributing to the movement of fatty tissues toward the mitochondria, where they are burned for energy.

ATP's dosing recommendations are listed below by weight; it's typically recommended that you take this supplement 45 minutes before a workout. I think this product could also be beneficial before any brain work: presentations, writing, studying or any other activity that increases the need for focus and recall.

> *Less than 150 pounds:* three capsules, 45 minutes before a workout or brain activity
> *150 to 200 pounds:* four capsules, 45 minutes before a workout or brain activity
> *More than 200 pounds:* five capsules, 45 minutes before a workout or brain activity

Boosting GH certainly promises many exciting benefits, including less abdominal fat, more muscle mass, fewer wrinkles, increased bone mass, improved cholesterol levels and stronger immune system function. But GH supplementation is no panacea for health. Neither is it free of associated risks. Abnormally high GH can raise blood sugar, contribute to insulin resistance, increase the risk of Type 2 diabetes and cause abnormal bone growth. New research also suggests that elevated IGF-1 may be a risk factor for certain types of malignancies, especially prostate cancer. So, as with almost all hormones, what we want is to increase levels to the correct amount steadily, not unleash a tidal wave.

Acetylcholine Basics

Acetylcholine is the neurotransmitter essential to the flow of communication between nerves and muscles. Movement, coordination and muscle tone are all influenced by acetylcholine, as it is the messenger molecule that allows your muscles to contract. Keeping acetylcholine levels high is one of the secrets of maintaining strong, healthy, metabolically-active muscle. I have included a discussion of acetylcholine in this chapter because it also stimulates GH release, which, as we've seen, improves tissue healing, promotes muscle growth, enhances skin tone and bone density and aids fat loss (especially the loss of abdominal fat).

The more we exercise, the more acetylcholine we use up. Athletes often have significant reductions in acetylcholine levels following strenuous activities such as running, cycling and swimming. We can, however, use natural supplements that stimulate the production of choline, the building block of acetylcholine, to vastly improve stamina and even reduce pre- and post-exercise fatigue.

How Acetylcholine Works for You

Along with muscle movement, REM (rapid eye movement) sleep, memory and mental alertness, concentration and learning are also linked to acetylcholine. Healthy digestion and regularity are also controlled by the chemical message acetylcholine delivers to smooth muscle cells along the digestive tract. Acetylcholine declines naturally with aging, and that decline is frequently combined with a decrease in physical activity. This may explain the constipation that plagues so many people later in life. This depletion is also thought to be one of the major culprits behind age-related memory loss, depression, mood changes, insomnia and Alzheimer's disease.

REM Sleep Aid

Ever wonder how the brain controls sleep—easily one of the body's most essential tasks? Researchers at the Massachusetts Institute of Technology

According to results in the September 2003 *Pharmacology Biochemistry and Behavior*, British scientists found that taking sage oil capsules significantly improved performance in a word-recall test in healthy adults. Finally, a scientific basis for the centuries-old idea of being "sage smart!"

Sage is currently being investigated as a potential treatment for Alzheimer's disease, after earlier research found that it inhibits an enzyme that breaks down acetylcholine. Alzheimer's— the most common form of dementia, affecting an estimated 10 million people worldwide—is accompanied by a drop in acetylcholine. Although further investigation is needed to determine why sage is so effective, researchers think it could be a combination of chemicals in the oil, that has an effect on acetylcholine and gives it antioxidant, estrogenic and anti-inflammatory properties, also considered valuable in Alzheimer's therapy.

Get "Sage Smart"

For the first time, researchers have proven that rosemary oil measurements in the blood correlate with improved cognitive performance, according to a study in *Therapeutic Advances in Psychopharmacology* (2012). The study was completed at the Brain Performance and Nutrition Research Center at Northumbria University and was designed to investigate the pharmacology of one of rosemary's main chemical constituents, called 1,8-cineole.

The investigators tested cognitive performance and mood in 20 subjects who inhaled certain amounts of rosemary essential oil. Using blood samples to detect the amount of 1,8-cineole that participants had absorbed, the researchers applied speed and accuracy tests and mood assessments to judge the rosemary oil's effects. And here's more proof that aromatherapy works: Higher concentrations of rosemary oil in the blood resulted in improved performance—in both speed and accuracy!

The chemical also appeared to have an effect on mood, although this was less pronounced. Contentment levels, however, did not appear to be correlated with the levels of 1,8-cineole in the blood, which is interesting, because it suggests that compounds given off by rosemary essential oil affect subjective state and cognitive performance through different brain pathways. In other words, different compounds contained within rosemary essential oil influence mood and cognitive performance.

Rosemary extracts can enter the bloodstream via the nasal or lung mucosa, and because they are small, fat-soluble organic molecules, they can easily cross the blood–brain barrier. Once there, they seem to inhibit the enzymes that break down acetylcholine, thereby increasing its levels, which are linked to enhanced memory.

and Massachusetts General Hospital have added to the mystery in a report published in the *Proceedings of the National Academy of Sciences* (January 2015): The activation of neurons that release acetylcholine is somehow able to induce REM sleep in an animal model.

Natural sleep is composed of alternating cycles of non-REM and REM sleep, each of which provides different benefits. Current sleep aids do not effectively restore normal sleep physiology or timing (lack of REM sleep is a well-documented side effect of sleep medications); as a result, they cannot replicate the important functions of natural sleep. Recognizing the link between acetylcholine and sleep could be a new means of treating insomnia and ineffective sleeping patterns in adults—without the side effects of traditional sleep medications.

Tips to Boost Acetylcholine

Clearly, keeping acetylcholine levels high is one of the secrets to maintaining strong, healthy, metabolically-active muscle—and your brain power too.

Foods and Habits

- **Exercise:** Yes, absolutely—but not too much, as it can cause overall depletion of acetylcholine without the proper nutritional precautions.
- **Nutrition:** Consume healthy fats and sources of choline such as lecithin, egg yolks, wheat germ, soybeans, organ meats (liver, kidney, etc.) and whole-wheat products.

Supplement Options

- **Acetyl-L-carnitine:** Acetyl-L-carnitine is a potent antioxidant for the brain and an anti-inflammatory that provides a source of the acetyl group needed to make acetylcholine, as well as L-carnitine, which assists with fat burning. Take 500 to 1,000 mg daily, preferably in the morning, before breakfast. Acetyl-L-carnitine is my favorite choice for boosting acetylcholine, aiding weight loss and slowing down the aging of the brain.
- **Phosphatidylcholine (PC; also called lecithin in some supplements):** PC provides choline, which is needed to make

acetylcholine. Take 1,200 to 2,400 mg daily with food. PC is my favorite choice for use during pregnancy. It supports development of the baby's brain and nervous system, and I swear the babies I see in my practice are smarter for it! For an intensive brain boost, I take four capsules of lecithin (from Biotics Research) as a source of acetylcholine before all speaking engagements or media appearances that require strong mental recall. I began taking this supplement after reading a study that proved it works when taken 90 minutes before intensive brain work, and I've seen the benefits first-hand.

- **DMAE:** Dimethylaminoethanol is an anti-inflammatory and antioxidant that increases the production of acetylcholine. It is useful for both cognitive function and improving muscle contractions. Take 100 to 300 mg daily with food. (As an aside, DMAE may also be used topically to improve skin tone and firmness.)
- **L-alpha-glycerylphosphorylcholine (alpha-GPC):** Glycerylphosphorylcholine plays an important role in the synthesis of acetylcholine—and it's a mouthful of a word! It maintains neurological health and may also help to enhance GH. The standard dose is one to two 500 mg capsules daily, away from food.
- **Rosemary and sage oils:** Both of these essential oils have been found to inhibit the breakdown of acetylcholine and therefore *increase* the activity of the hormone, when taken orally or inhaled via essential aromatic oils before activities that test recall. I have two options for you: Candibactin-AR (Metagenics) or Neuroloft (North American Herb and Spice). Either should be taken as a dose of two to four capsules daily, with food.

GH is kind of like the body's mission control: It affects almost every cell, allowing tissue to repair and muscle to build. It supports bone density and a healthy body composition. And like all good rechargers, it does some of its best work when you're asleep. Acetylcholine, on the other hand, is your communication center: It allows your nerves and muscles to talk to each other. That's hugely important for things like REM sleep, memory and mental capacities like alertness, concentration and learning. So, whether your body needs to recharge more fully or be a better communicator, you've now got the tools to support it. Another one of those tools comes, surprisingly, right from your fat cells.

A HORMONE BOOST REAL-LIFE SUCCESS STORY

THE CLIENT: Linda V.

DETAILS: Female, 47

BODY COMPOSITION RESULTS (FROM SCALE AND BODY FAT/ MUSCLE MASS VIA BIO-IMPEDANCE TESTING)

MEASUREMENT	BEFORE	AFTER	TOTAL LOSS/GAIN
Weight (lb.)	146	137	(-) 9
Lean Body Mass (lb.)	108.0	108.5	(+) 0.5
Fat Mass (lb.)	38	28.5	(-) 9.5
Basal Metabolic Rate (calories/day)	1,529 calories	1,540 calories	(+) 11

Linda's initial complaints on her intake form were as follows:
- Don't sleep solidly throughout the night
- Fatigued most of the time
- Low energy
- Can be moody
- My motivation is affected

- Sluggish digestion due to constipation
- PMS

After following the Hormone Boost plan, this is what Linda reported:
- Sleeping more solidly
- Energy and stress adaptation ability much improved
- Mood more stable—and fewer "lows," even though handling a lot with family
- Workouts and drive much stronger
- Constipation a non-issue and no abdominal bloating
- No more PMS—including breast pain, cramping and headaches!

What an amazing transformation. All this *and* she lost almost 10 pounds of fat and gained half a pound of muscle. Her underactive thyroid function also dramatically improved: Her TSH went from 10.97 (the ideal is less than 2) to 3.14 in just four weeks. Awesome!

CHAPTER 5

FAT-LOSS HORMONE #5:
ANY WAY YOU ADD IT UP, ADIPONECTIN SUBTRACTS FAT

Nothing is impossible; the word itself says, "I'm possible."

AUDREY HEPBURN, actress

The benefit of adiponectin simply seems too good to be true—essentially, it burns fat. In some animal testing models, this fantastic advantage appeared without a coinciding increase in hunger. The biggest benefits of this fat-burning hormone, however, may prove to go well beyond your belly, hips and thighs.

Adiponectin Basics

Adiponectin is a hormone produced in and sent out from our fat cells. The appropriate amounts of adiponectin can decrease inflammation and fuel fat loss. Even though it's produced by our fat cells, it actually helps us lose fat by improving our insulin sensitivity. Think of adiponectin as the fat factor that ironically leads to its own demise; it's produced by your fat but helps to burn it up!

Adiponectin is currently being studied as a possible cure for cardiovascular disease and a diabetes treatment. When injected into test subjects, it has been found to drastically increase insulin sensitivity, relax blood vessels and directly reduce inflammation within the cardiovascular system. Amazingly, should you suffer the misfortune of having a heart attack, your body releases huge amounts of adiponectin in a frantic attempt to quickly heal the damage.

How Adiponectin Works for You

Adiponectin was first described relatively recently, in 1995, and I've yet to find mention of a downside to its abundance. It seems nothing but good things come from the effects of this metabolic hormone. The March 2016 issue of the *Journal of Molecular Cell Biology* summarized adiponectin's benefits from hundreds of studies over the past two decades, linking it to improvements in obesity, diabetes, inflammation, atherosclerosis and cardiovascular disease.

If all this weren't enough, adiponectin has been shown to induce apoptosis (intentional, programmed cell death) in certain types of cancers. This protective benefit is easier to get than you think, as you'll see from my more in-depth discussion of food choices and exercise habits in this chapter. For instance, women were able to increase their levels of adiponectin simply by increasing the quantity of tomatoes in their diet. Impressive! So, what else can adiponectin do for you?

Insulin-Sensitizing and Fat-Burning Friend

Like adiponectin, leptin—a fat cell–produced hormone that regulates appetite and energy expenditure—is also a fat-loss friend. Adiponectin and leptin work in opposition to resistin, a hormone that contributes to fat gain by directly causing insulin resistance in the liver and muscle cells. While adiponectin aids fat burning, resistin actually fuels the creation of more fat from fat.

Insulin signals the body to either store energy as fat or burn it as fuel. Adiponectin levels may be a predictor of insulin resistance, according to a study published in the March 2011 *European Journal of Clinical Nutrition*. Researchers evaluated the activities of adiponectin, leptin and fatty acid composition within the cell membranes that may be involved in insulin resistance. Participants with diabetes took a glucose tolerance test, that assessed glucose measurements, HbA1c (a measure of blood sugar over several months prior to the test), insulin, leptin, adiponectin and red blood cell membrane composition. Participants with impaired glucose tolerance showed lower levels of essential fatty acids in their red blood cell membranes, which correlated with lower levels of adiponectin and higher levels of insulin and insulin resistance.

To give you an idea of how important this hormone is, consider this: Some animal models have shown a reversal of insulin resistance with adiponectin infusions. Since high levels of adiponectin correspond with improved insulin sensitivity, this in turn assists in the metabolizing of carbohydrates. The reality is, someone who is insulin resistant is also often carb sensitive and may have difficulty processing carbohydrates (this is the basis of my book *The Carb Sensitivity Program*).

So it seems that the higher your adiponectin levels, the greater your energy/caloric expenditure (that is, the more calories you burn, even at rest). Adiponectin increases fatty acid oxidation in muscle cells; simply put, it burns more fat. It also increases insulin sensitivity, improves glucose tolerance and inhibits inflammation, and all three help you get and stay slim.

Compared to a low-fat diet, a very-low-carb diet yielded better fat loss and improved adiponectin levels, according to researchers at the University of Cincinnati (2011). If someone is insulin resistant, then reducing carbs—or, more particularly, determining the right carbs for their physiology—reduces excess insulin and, in turn, increases the presence of fat-burning hormones such as adiponectin. A low-carb diet alone, however, won't solely improve adiponectin status, since there are many other factors in play. Incorporating the right type of healthy fats (i.e., monounsaturated fats, like those in olive oil, nuts, etc.), ample protein, walking and strength training all work together to boost adiponectin levels.

Anti-aging Ace

Both humans and mice that manage to live to a ripe old age show a clear change in their glucose metabolism, according to a study by the American Society for Biochemistry and Molecular Biology (November 2007). Terry Combs and his colleagues reported that changes in metabolism can indeed increase longevity; they discovered that long-lived mice burn less glucose and more fatty acids during periods of fasting and, as a result, produce fewer free radicals.

The key to this switch may be fasting—which we've already discussed for its growth hormone benefits—and its associated adiponectin boost. Researchers found that Snell mice had three times as much adiponectin in their blood as control mice. The Snell mice also had fewer triglycerides in their cells, indicative of higher fat metabolism. I'm a huge animal lover, and I love my dog, Walter, so much that I reflect on calorie-restriction studies of monkeys—and this new one on Snell mice—and think he should do the Hormone Boost fast day so I can have him with me as long as possible!

A Closer Look

So now you know: Adiponectin, in a nutshell, is amazing. As I said at the beginning of this chapter, however, it's also relatively new to the field of weight loss and hormonal health. This book just might be the first time many of you have heard of this fat-busting friend. For this reason and more, it's worth a more in-depth look at the foods and habits you can use to get your adiponectin boost.

Healthy Fats Help

Amazingly, researchers have found that intake of monounsaturated fats such as fish oil boosts levels of adiponectin by 14 to 60 percent. This may be explained in part by research in *Diabetes Care* (July 2007) that found that replacing saturated fat with monounsaturated fat resulted in increases in fasting adiponectin levels. Along with being good for your heart, monounsaturated fats are also ideal for maintaining a lean body. Replacing saturated fat with monoun-saturated fat (reducing saturated fat from 23 percent to 9 percent of caloric intake) increased fasting adiponectin levels.

Safflower oil has also been shown to trigger the production of adiponectin, which assists in the catabolism of fatty acids. In the presence of safflower oil, adiponectin production increases up to 20 percent more than usual. In fact, research from Ohio State University (2011) shows that 1.5 tablespoons of safflower oil—naturally high in an omega-6 compound known as linolenic acid—a day can lower cholesterol, balance blood sugar levels and reduce trunk fat in postmenopausal women, by virtue of its positive effects on adiponectin levels. In the study, 16 weeks of supplementation with this super-oil also had another, unanticipated side effect: increased muscle tissue. As a bonus, you can add a little safflower oil to your conditioner to moisturize your hair and nourish hair follicles. I recommend getting your health-promoting dose of this oil by consuming four capsules per day of conjugated linoleic acid (CLA) derived from safflower oil (check out Clear CLA; it's the most effective form of CLA I have found to date).

A diet rich in olive oil not only aids appetite control and prevents belly fat accumulation, it also guards against the insulin resistance and drop in adiponectin typically seen in people who eat a high-carbohydrate diet (which is, unfortunately, far too many of us). According to a study in the *Journal of the American College of Nutrition* (October 2007), consuming olive oil at breakfast is especially effective in this regard.

So, making the dietary switch to more monounsaturated fats appears to lead to a redistribution of body fat away from the abdomen. This is fantastic, considering that your total calorie intake can remain unchanged. Monounsaturated fats improve glucose utilization and insulin sensitivity. And even better news—these are the tastiest fats to eat! They include avocados, nuts, olive oil and olives. If you're getting sick of topping your salads with olive oil, try using avocado oil or macadamia nut oil (which can also be used when cooking at high heat) for the same hormone benefits and different taste experiences.

Fill Up on Fiber

Good old fiber still seems to be a time-tested leader in the weight-loss field—but now we have cutting-edge evidence to explain its dominance. Researchers have found that adding fiber to the diet increased adiponectin levels by as much as 115 percent! Fiber also stabilizes glucose levels and reduces the glycemic impact of meals (i.e., the blood-sugar spike after you eat), which improves insulin sensitivity. I can't say enough about getting your 35 g of fiber per day. It's so simple, but the influences on your fat loss and hormonal balance are really profound.

All About Exercise

Adiponectin plays an important role in the energetic capacity of skeletal muscle, according to a study in the July 2006 issue of *Cell Metabolism*. There's evidence (in both people and mice) linking low adiponectin levels to insulin resistance and reductions in the number of cellular "power plants," called mitochondria, in skeletal muscle. Therapies designed to boost the adiponectin signal might therefore prove beneficial for the treatment of insulin resistance and diabetes. Mitochondria utilize nutrient components, including fats and carbohydrates, to generate usable energy, and the number of mitochondria influences the way that muscles function. People who exercise regularly will have more mitochondria in their muscles than those who are sedentary.

Earlier studies found that obese individuals and those with Type 2 diabetes have reduced adiponectin concentrations. To counteract this, participants were asked to perform moderate exercise daily. This raised levels of the hormone by up to 48 percent! To experience an increase in adiponectin, this research suggests, you need moderate exercise at least three times a week. The elevation in adiponectin levels occurs for 24 to 72 hours—which explains my inspiration to suggest walking at least three times per week as part of the Hormone Boost workout.

As we age, our risk for insulin resistance increases. We're more prone to belly fat and reduced lean muscle mass, which leaves us burning fewer calories than we did in our more youthful days. The more fat tissue you have, the lower your adiponectin levels, which perpetuates the cycle of insulin resistance and belly fat. But there's good news for yogis and you alike—yoga, like walking, has been shown to reverse this cycle in postmenopausal women, because yoga improves adiponectin, cholesterol levels and metabolic syndrome risk factors.

Don't Kick Your Coffee Habit

Regular coffee consumption has been linked to an increase in adiponectin levels and a reduction in pro-inflammatory cytokines, which could boost weight loss and reduce inflammation levels. In fact, habitual coffee consumption was associated with high adiponectin levels in a study published in the *European Journal of Nutrition* (June 2011) involving Japanese males. And while green tea is often touted as a healthier form of caffeine intake, coffee was demonstrably more successful than green tea in boosting adiponectin. The Hormone Boost recommends organic, fair-trade coffee; you can enjoy a cup early in the day or before a workout for best results.

Top Up the Turmeric

Turmeric (also known as curcumin) fights inflammation, which, at high levels, contributes to weight gain. As well as working at the fat-cell level, turmeric increases adiponectin production and improves insulin sensitivity. It works by reducing the hormones in your fat cells that cause inflammation (primarily resistin and leptin) and it boosts adiponectin, which helps control appetite. If you prefer supplements, take one to two capsules on an empty stomach (30 minutes before a meal or two hours after). If you experience heartburn, take it with food instead.

Revel in Red Wine

Raise your glass if you are healthy in all the right ways! Resveratrol, a compound in grapes, displays antioxidant and other positive properties. A 2011 study in the *Journal of Biological Chemistry* by researchers at the University of Texas Health Science Center at San Antonio describes one way that resveratrol exerts these beneficial health effects: It stimulates the expression of adiponectin. Both adiponectin and resveratrol display anti-obesity, anti–insulin resistance and anti-aging properties. I take two capsules of Resveratrim (my Clear Medicine highly absorbable and bioactive resveratrol supplement) every morning.

Consume Your Carbs at Dinner

Yes, you read that correctly: Carbs in the evening are actually good for you! According to a 2012 research study completed at the Hebrew University of Jerusalem, an experimental diet with carbohydrates eaten mostly at dinner, rather than during the day, seems to benefit people suffering from severe and morbid obesity. This diet seems to influence the secretion patterns of the hormones responsible for hunger and satiety, as well as the hormones associated with metabolic syndrome, including a boost in the daytime production of adiponectin. But there was another important discovery that came from this study. These effects appeared to help dieters persist over the long run; the study lasted six months and the participants stuck with it. This suggests that there is an advantage to concentrating carbohydrate intake in the evening, a benefit that could translate to all of us, but especially to people at risk of developing diabetes or cardiovascular disease due to obesity.

You Say Tomato, I Say Yes!

A tomato-rich diet may help protect at-risk postmenopausal women from breast cancer, according to new research in the Endocrine Society's *Journal of Clinical Endocrinology & Metabolism* (December 2013). Eating a diet high in tomatoes had a positive effect on the level of hormones that play a role in regulating fat and sugar metabolism, particularly adiponectin.

The study assessed the effects of both tomato-rich and soy-rich diets in a collection of 70 postmenopausal women. For 10 weeks the women ate tomato products containing at least 25 mg of lycopene daily. For a separate 10-week period, the participants consumed at least 40 g of soy protein daily. Before each test period began, the women were instructed to abstain from eating both tomato and soy products for two weeks. We know that eating fruits and vegetables rich in essential nutrients, vitamins, minerals and phytochemicals such as lycopene conveys significant benefits. Based on this data, regular consumption of at least the daily recommended servings of fruits and vegetables would promote breast cancer prevention in an at-risk population.

When they followed the tomato-rich diet, participants' levels of adiponectin climbed 9 percent. Interestingly, the soy diet was linked to a *reduction* in participants' adiponectin levels. Researchers originally theorized that a diet containing large amounts of soy could be part of the reason why Asian women have lower rates of breast cancer than women in the United States, but any beneficial effect may be limited to certain ethnic groups. Regardless, including tomatoes in your diet contributes to healthy adiponectin levels.

Give Me an Adiponectin Boost—Fast!

Intermittent fasting is all the rage—but it turns out to be more than just a diet trend. A scientific review in the *British Journal of Diabetes and Vascular Disease* suggests that fasting diets may also help those with diabetes and cardiovascular disease.

Intermittent fasting—fasting on a given number of consecutive or alternate days—has recently been hailed as a path to weight loss and lowered cardiovascular risk. A team led by Dr. James Brown from Aston University (April 2013) evaluated the various approaches to intermittent fasting in scientific literature. They searched specifically for the advantages and limitations of treating obesity and Type 2 diabetes using fasting diets. The basic format of intermittent fasting is to alternate days eating "normally" with days when calorie consumption is restricted. This can be done either on alternate days (day 1: eat normally; day 2: restrict) or by establishing two days within each week as fasting days. These types of intermittent fasting have been shown in trials to be *as effective as* or *more effective than* counting calories every day to lose weight. Evidence from clinical trials shows that fasting can limit inflammation, improve levels of sugars and fats in circulation by impacting adiponectin and reduce blood pressure.

Tips for an Adiponectin Boost

Now that you have all the information you need about the wonders of adiponectin, here's a summary of how best to get your boost of this super-helpful hormone.

Foods and Habits

- **General:** Dietary management is considered a great means of modulating adiponectin levels. The suggestions here are summarized from Medline clinical trials.
  > Daily intake of fish or omega-3 supplementation increased adiponectin levels by 14 to 60 percent.
  > Weight loss achieved with a low-caloric diet plus exercise increased adiponectin levels in the range of 18 to 48 percent.
  > A 60 to 115 percent increase in adiponectin levels was obtained with fiber supplementation. Get fiber four times per day—eating some at every meal.

- **Exercise:** We've seen that exercise increases adiponectin levels; it seems that how much correlates to fat levels in the body. This is good news—the bigger your fat cells, the greater effect exercise will have. It doesn't seem as if the particular type of exercises matters; rather, the key is to *move more*. Research shows that people who move more have higher levels of adiponectin. The best exercise for adiponectin looks, in fact, much like the Hormone Boost workout:
  - Walk at least three times per week.
  - Do yoga one to two times per week.
  - Strength-train two to three times per week.
- **Nutrition:**
  - Adiponectin is boosted by the monounsaturated fats found in avocados, olives and olive oil, macadamia nuts and sesame oil.
  - Consume blueberries daily as your fruit selection. The cyanidin 3-glucoside antioxidant in blueberries causes anti-obesity activities within the fat cell, one of which is increasing adiponectin release and adiponectin gene expression.
  - Include tomato juice and cooked tomatoes in your diet daily.
  - Consume your starchy carbs at dinner—no other times during the day.
  - Drink coffee, especially before a workout or in the morning, but only one cup per day.
- **Do the Hormone Boost fasting day:** Our fasting bodies change how they select which fuel to burn, improving metabolism and reducing oxidative stress. Today's intermittent fasting regimens are easier to stick to, and they're proven to help excess pounds melt away. The benefits of fasting may be due in part to the increase of adiponectin it stimulates. Tips for the intermittent fasting day are outlined

for you in the nutrition plan of the Hormone Boost, in Chapter 10.

Supplement Options

Antioxidants have a powerful effect on adipokines, especially adiponectin. These are the antioxidants that stand out:

- **Green coffee bean extract:** Chances are you've heard the buzz about this supplement. If not, it certainly deserves your attention now. Here's the surprising skinny on green coffee bean: Scientists have shown that this product can produce a substantial decrease in body weight in a relatively short period of time. Their study involved 16 overweight or obese individuals who took a low-dose green coffee bean extract, a high-dose coffee bean extract or a placebo 30 minutes before a meal, without changing their exercise or nutrition habits. Participants lost an average of 17 pounds during the 22 weeks of the study, which included an average 10.5 percent decrease in overall body weight and a 16 percent decrease in body fat. An even more interesting note: a daily intake of 2,400 calories was maintained during the study, which is *not* a low-calorie diet by any means. In another study, published in *Phytothérapie* (2006), 400 mg of green coffee bean daily caused fat loss in volunteers. Clear Vive provides a great source of coffee bean extract—pop one capsule before a workout and you won't believe how much energy you feel!
- **Turmeric (curcumin):** Turmeric fights inflammation at the fat-cell level while also increasing adiponectin production. Add the spice to your foods or take two to three capsules daily, away from food.
- **Zinc:** The level of adiponectin increased significantly in subjects who received 50 mg of zinc compared to a control group, according to a study published in the *Iranian Journal of*

Diabetes and Obesity (June 2012). Take 30 to 50 mg of zinc for a maximum of 12 weeks only, then reduce the dose or switch to a multivitamin containing zinc.

- **Green tea:** According to a study in the May 2015 issue of *Clinical Nutrition*, 12 weeks of treatment with high-dose green tea extract resulted in significant weight loss, reduced waist circumference, and a consistent decrease in total cholesterol and LDL plasma levels—without any side effects or adverse effects in women with central obesity. The mechanism driving these benefits of high-dose green tea extract is most likely associated with a reduction in secretion of the hunger hormone ghrelin and an increase in adiponectin levels. One hundred and fifteen women were given 856.8 mg of EGCG (green tea extract) per day. After 12 weeks, the average weight loss was about 25 pounds, with no side effects. Amazing! This is the dosage you need to aim for daily.

- **Resveratrol:** Resveratrol is known to boost adiponectin and reduce inflammation. My Resveratrim is methylated resveratrol, which means it is eight times more active in your body. Take two capsules daily upon rising or in a divided dose— one in the morning and one mid-afternoon.

- **Adipolitik (from ATP Labs):** You can look for a product that contains a combination of many of these ingredients, such as Adipolitik. Take four capsules daily, preferably away from food. Then add zinc and resveratrol separately if you wish to complete your prescription for an adiponectin boost.

You can't get away from insulin sensitivity these days—sugars seem like they're hidden *everywhere*. Having adiponectin as one of the tools in your Hormone Boost kit will help balance your insulin. Even better, though, is that the higher your levels are (i.e., the more you follow the suggestions above), the more efficiently you will burn calories, even at rest! And to ensure that your body is using the right fuel to burn those calories, you'll want to tap glucagon for support.

A HORMONE BOOST REAL-LIFE SUCCESS STORY

THE CLIENT: Joanna B.

DETAILS: Female, 34

BODY COMPOSITION RESULTS (FROM SCALE AND BODY FAT/ MUSCLE MASS VIA BIO-IMPEDANCE TESTING)

MEASUREMENT	BEFORE	AFTER	TOTAL LOSS/GAIN
Weight (lb.)	139	129	(-) 10
Lean Body Mass (lb.)	99.0	99.5	(+) 0.5
Fat Mass (lb.)	40	29.5	(-) 10.5
Basal Metabolic Rate (calories/day)	1,401 calories	1,407 calories	(+) 6

Joanna is one of three women I worked with for six weeks for a special episode of the *Marilyn Denis Show* that was all about losing belly fat, especially the dreaded and stubborn last 10 pounds. She is a working mom of two—a stressed-out, burned-out, multitasking superwoman. I am sure you know the type! Within just four days on the program, her energy was dramatically better and her cravings were gone. By the end of the six weeks, she had lost 10.5 pounds of fat and gained 0.5 pound of muscle. She also lost five inches off her belly!

You can watch the show at www.marilyn.ca/mobile/Segment? segid=109608.

CHAPTER 6

FAT-LOSS HORMONE #6:
GO, GO, GLUCAGON!

What you do speaks so loudly that
I cannot hear what you say.

RALPH WALDO EMERSON

It's all about balance. Those of you who have read *The Hormone Diet* and *The Supercharged Hormone Diet* know that our goal must be not only weight loss but also *hormonal balance*. In all of my previous books, you also heard me say that a reduction in insulin is essential to achieving greater fat loss and preserving the metabolically active muscle tissue we need to burn calories more efficiently at all times, even at rest. Muscle tissue is for improving insulin sensitivity and fueling your fat-burning furnace.

There is a direct relationship among our carbohydrate intake, blood sugar balance and insulin levels. Carbs are broken down into sugar, the sugar goes into the bloodstream, and insulin is released to then carry the sugar into our cells. So carbs spike the one hormone that tells our body to store energy as fat—insulin. Nonetheless, no matter what popular diet books say, cutting out carbs completely is not a good weight-loss strategy. When we eliminate carbs, we take away one of the body's primary fuel sources—and create a negative hormonal chain reaction.

For instance, a total lack of carbs can cause physical stress and elevate levels of the stress hormone cortisol, which can in turn lead to loss of muscle tissue and an increase in abdominal fat. Without carbs, testosterone plummets, leaving our libido flat and our muscles depleted. At the same time, our happy hormone, serotonin, takes a dip, and we experience cravings, bingeing, depression and sleep disruption. No wonder a no-carb diet is associated with irritability, fatigue and poor performance! It's also unsustainable. Our body naturally puts up a fight when we restrict carbs. Our stress- and appetite-boosting hormones cause us to overeat, and our sinking thyroid hormones put the brakes on our metabolism—certainly not an ideal health-and-wellness scenario.

Unfortunately, the majority of us have far too much insulin, due to choosing the wrong carbs and dietary and lifestyle habits. I can assure you that the only way to stop this cycle and repair your metabolism is by choosing the right types and amounts of carbohydrates, as well as the right times to ingest them. This will stabilize blood sugar and reduce insulin release, and it will do so by building more muscle, the largest tissues in the body where insulin does its work. But there is another reason these actions have such terrific benefits— they also stimulate the last of the six fat-loss hormones: glucagon.

Glucagon Basics

Insulin lowers our blood sugar by transporting glucose from the bloodstream into liver cells, muscle cells and fat cells for storage as glycogen or fat. Glucagon works in direct opposition—it raises blood sugar by breaking down stored glycogen and fat. When we exercise, consume protein or experience a dip in blood sugar, glucagon kicks in to aid fat loss by instructing the body to use stored fat and sugars for fuel. Glucagon release is inhibited, however, when high amounts of sugar and insulin are present in our bloodstream.

Since protein consumption stimulates glucagon activity, eating substantial amounts of meat, dairy, soy or fish seems like a great approach to weight loss, right? Not necessarily. Your body much prefers carbohydrates over protein for use as an energy source. In fact, we *want* the body to choose sugar over protein for fuel, because the latter process can break down muscle. Excess glucagon can also destroy the precious muscle tissue we work so hard to build and maintain.

The key to maintaining a stable blood sugar level while also preventing breakdown of muscle tissue is to balance protein consumption with low-glycemic carbohydrates such as fruits, vegetables, whole-grain breads and grains like quinoa—carbohydrates that limit insulin secretion. This combination of foods will promote glucagon release while also providing your body with sufficient fuel. If you consume too many carbohydrates or fail to eat enough protein, you will not benefit from the fat-burning effects of glucagon.

The Glycemic Index and Its Relationship to Glucagon

So you want to shed a few pounds? Eating a "balanced" diet isn't always enough, as evidenced by the myriad of diet books that have popped up (and continue to pop up!) over the years, offering countless pages of advice on how to "get over the hump" and lose that weight. Much has been written about the value of low-carb diets, high-protein diets, complex carbohydrates and the glycemic index. Despite all this information, or perhaps because of it, many of us are left feeling confused about what to eat.

While we readily think of bread, pasta, rice, cereals, cookies, cakes, pastries, chips, pretzels and potatoes as the usual suspects when it comes to carb or "starch" sources, most of my patients are surprised to learn that vegetables, fruits and legumes (beans) are also sources of carbs. But by far the sneakiest of all carbs are the plethora of sometimes hidden sugars that make their way into common food items: syrups, jams, jellies, juices, candies, chocolate milk, flavored yogurts, flavored waters (flat or sparkling), sodas, sauces, energy drinks, energy bars, specialty coffees, granola and other cereals or granola bars. All carbs, regardless of their form, eventually become sugar (also known as glucose) in our bloodstream.

Essentially there are two types of carbs, and what differentiates the two is the rate at which the body converts them into glucose. The so-called "good" carbs, or complex carbs, are converted into sugar in much smaller amounts and at a much slower rate than their not-so-good counterparts. Complex carbs contain more fiber than their bad cousins and, as a result, spark less of an insulin release. The "bad carbs" initiate a fast and furious rush of sugar into the bloodstream, a situation that can result in mood swings, cravings, fatigue and even headaches.

We can differentiate good carbs from bad by looking at the glycemic index (GI). The GI is the measurement of how quickly a food ends up as sugar in your bloodstream after consumption. High-glycemic foods such as white pasta, white rice, potato chips, pastries, cookies, candies, muffins, sodas, bagels and white potatoes are broken down rapidly, and these foods are usually also low in fiber. As a result, they cause a huge influx of sugar into our bloodstream, followed by *loads* of insulin.

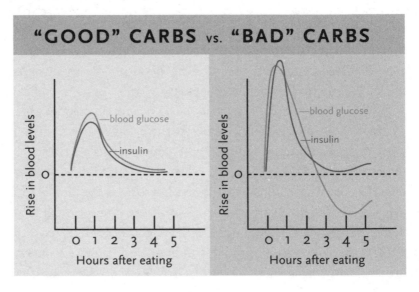

On the other hand, low-glycemic carbohydrates such as berries, green vegetables and legumes are broken down slowly, allowing sugar to trickle gradually into the bloodstream, thereby limiting insulin release. Low-glycemic carbohydrates typically have a glycemic index of less than 55 and, as mentioned earlier, tend to be higher in fiber. Moderate-GI foods are in the range of 55 to 70; high-GI foods are greater than 70. So remember, low = slow = go for it, in most cases—*if* your insulin metabolism is healthy.

The glycemic load (GL) is a newer measure that builds upon the principles of the glycemic index. The GL provides an idea of the *total* glycemic response to a food or meal (how quickly and how much your blood sugar increases after the item is ingested); it also takes into consideration the amount of carbohydrate per serving. On this scale, a low glycemic load is below 10. While low-glycemic carbohydrates always have a low glycemic load, some foods with a high glycemic index actually have a *low glycemic load*. Take carrots: They have a high glycemic index, which has prompted most weight-loss diets to recommend avoiding them. But a single serving of carrots actually has a relatively low amount of carbohydrate. As a result, carrots have a low glycemic load, which in fact makes them a *good* choice for those who practice carb-conscious eating habits.

The idea of consuming low-glycemic-load carbohydrates together with lean sources of protein and healthy fats formed the foundation of my first book, *The Hormone Diet*. Step 2—in which I recommend one serving of grains or starchy vegetables (such as sweet potato), one serving of legumes, two of fruit, unlimited non-starchy veggies and one serving of nuts as the daily sources of carbohydrates—taught readers how to eat for hormonal balance. This way of eating certainly represents a balanced, carb-conscious diet (by no means a no-carb diet), yet a small percentage of patients failed to continue losing weight. The question I had to ask was why, especially since all the carbs I recommended were healthy, low-GI carbs. Thus began my latest research into the net carb content of my recommendations.

When you read nutrition labels, you see that the total amount of carbohydrate is composed mainly of fiber and sugar. "Net carbs" refers to the carbs that will have an impact on your blood sugar and insulin levels—not the total carbs in a serving. It may sound complicated, but discovering a food's net carb content is actually very simple: Look for the carb total on the label, then subtract the fiber. The remaining carbs are the ones that affect your blood sugar—also called "impact carbs." For example, the label on a box of crackers might say that a serving includes 20 g of carbohydrates along with 6 g of fiber. This means that the product's net carb content is 14 g.

My investigation into net carbs led to two revelations. First, I was shocked to discover such a wide variation in the net carb content of healthy, low-GI carbs. I could not believe, for example, that sweet potato has almost 20 g more net carbs than squash! This would certainly have an impact on one's potential for achieving weight loss while still feeling satisfied, balanced and happy. Second, I realized that each individual's tolerance for carbs varies. I noticed that some people appeared to have an insulin spike even with a small amount of healthy, low-GI carbs, carbs that *should* have allowed them to avoid the blood-sugar spike and subsequent insulin surge that can fuel weight gain.

It is difficult, if not impossible, to predict the blood-glucose reaction of any one person to a certain carbohydrate, even when net carb content is carefully evaluated. Healthy, metabolically fit people who do not have a problem processing glucose will naturally have less of a reaction than those who are prediabetic or beginning to develop a mild blood-sugar and insulin imbalance. Prediabetics still have a blood sugar reading within the normal range, but their insulin levels are higher than normal. These are the people most likely to respond well to a low-carb or carb-conscious diet.

The Next Step in Indexes: The Insulin Index

A group of researchers decided to test the insulin response to foods, as insulin, not the glycemic index, is the true driver of obesity. An insulin index of 38 common foods can be found in the November 1997 issue of the *American Journal of Clinical Nutrition*. The portion size of each food tested contained 240 calories, and each food was given a percentage score relative to white bread, which was used as a reference at 100 percent.

Not surprisingly, the amounts of total carbohydrate and sugar in foods were positively related to their insulin index, whereas fat and protein contents were inversely related. This is to say that the more carbohydrate and sugar a food contained, the more insulin was released; but the more fat and protein, the less insulin was released. In general, the insulin index is similar to the glycemic index, but there are a few anomalies. Some protein-rich foods and bakery products—which were rich in fat and refined carbohydrates—actually have a higher insulin index than glycemic index.

INSULIN INDEX VS. GLYCEMIC INDEX OF 38 FOODS

FOOD	GLYCEMIC SCORE	INSULIN SCORE
BREAKFAST CEREALS		
All-Bran	40	32
Oatmeal	60	40
Muesli	60	40
Special K	70	66
Honey Smacks	60	67
Sustain	66	71
Cornflakes	76	75
CARBOHYDRATE-RICH FOODS		
White pasta	46	40
Brown pasta	68	40
Grain (rye) bread	60	56
Brown rice	104	62

FOOD	GLYCEMIC SCORE	INSULIN SCORE
French fries	71	74
White rice	110	79
Whole-wheat bread	97	96
White bread	100	100
Potatoes	141	121
PROTEIN-RICH FOODS		
Eggs	42	31
Cheese	55	45
Beef	21	51
Lentils	62	58
Fish	28	59
Baked beans	114	120
FRUIT		
Apples	50	59
Oranges	39	60
Bananas	79	81
Grapes	74	82
SNACKS AND SWEETS		
Peanuts	12	20
Popcorn	62	54
Potato chips	52	61
Ice cream	70	89
Yogurt	62	115
Mars bar	79	112
Jelly beans	118	160
BAKERY PRODUCTS		
Doughnuts	63	74
Croissants	74	79
Cakes	56	82
Crackers	118	87
Cookies	74	92

SOURCE: www.mendosa.com/insulin_index.htm

So this is where things get confusing: Protein, it turns out, is surprisingly potent at stimulating insulin. Beef and fish, for instance, have virtually no effect on blood glucose levels, yet they stimulate insulin almost as much as most cereals.

The reality is that insulin responses to foods varies greatly from person to person—depending on an individual's metabolic fitness and their dietary habits. For instance, some of the factors suspected or shown to affect insulin secretion include the presence of dietary fiber, the form of the food (whole foods), how it is cooked (e.g., pasta cooked al dente causes less insulin than if cooked soft), the addition of vinegar (acetic acid), and the addition of spices such as chili peppers (capsaicin). Meanwhile, the amount of sleep, stress and exercise dictates metabolic fitness (i.e., insulin sensitivity) and also, ultimately, subsequent insulin release.

But how is the insulin release from protein-rich and dairy foods possible? Well, it's the reason I quit lattes years ago; milk and most milk products contain a lot of sugar (lactose), so it makes sense that their insulin index would be higher and that they are contraindicated for insulin-resistant individuals. But why the insulin spike with beef and fish, when they contain no carbohydrates?

Even though carbohydrates are the major macronutrient from an insulin perspective, certain amino acids are capable of provoking an insulin surge as well, such as the branched-chain amino acid (BCAA) leucine. We know from studies that insulin is released and increases in the blood following a meal containing significant amounts of protein-containing leucine. This is a beneficial reaction, as insulin helps to draw the amino acids into the muscle from the bloodstream in order to stimulate new growth and repair.

During catabolic periods, such as fasting or energy restriction, supplementing with leucine or a complete mixture of the three BCAAs—leucine, isoleucine and valine—stimulates muscle protein synthesis. Likewise, leucine supplementation stimulates the recovery of muscle protein synthesis after exercise. By contrast, an insulin surge provoked by excess sugars will pull carbohydrates into the muscle. But when muscle glycogen levels are full, the excess sugar must be converted into body fat.

There is another important difference between carbs and protein and their influence on insulin release. Unlike carbohydrates, protein foods also cause the pancreas to secrete glucagon. At the beginning of this chapter, I mentioned that glucagon opposes some of the potentially harmful effects of insulin. As a result, although high-protein foods can cause a significant insulin release, they rarely have the same blood-sugar-roller-coaster, hunger-inducing effects that high-carbohydrate foods do.

How Glucagon Works for You

While too much insulin makes you feel hungry and pack on the pounds, glucagon can be your secret weapon for counteracting insulin's nasty effects. Here's how to make sure it's working for you:

Blood Glucose Regulator

Glucagon's role in the body is to prevent blood glucose levels from dropping too low. To do this, it acts on the liver in several ways:

- It stimulates the conversion of glycogen stored in the liver to glucose, which can be released into the bloodstream. This process is called *glycogenolysis*.
- It promotes the production of glucose from amino acid molecules. This process is called *gluconeogenesis*.
- It reduces glucose consumption by the liver, so that as much glucose as possible can be secreted into the bloodstream to maintain blood glucose levels.
- Glucagon also acts on fat (adipose) tissue to stimulate the breakdown and movement of fat stores into the bloodstream.

Because of its direct involvement in the regulation of blood sugar balance, glucagon is naturally linked to avoiding weight gain, metabolic syndrome and diabetes.

Appetite Suppressor

Eating a meal with a low GI increases gut hormone production, which in turn leads to appetite suppression and feeling full. Information presented by King's College London researchers at a Society for Endocrinology BES meeting in Harrogate (March 2009) revealed the effects of a low- versus high-GI meal on gut hormone levels. It was one of the first studies to explore how a low-GI meal produces satiety; it takes longer to digest and releases sugar into the bloodstream more slowly than a high-GI meal. It now appears that glucagon-like peptide-1 (GLP-1), a hormone produced by the gut, causes a feeling of fullness and the suppression of appetite. Volunteers who ate a low-GI breakfast had 20 percent higher blood plasma levels of GLP-1 and 38 percent lower insulin levels, compared to those who had consumed a high-GI breakfast.

Diabetes Buster?

A new treatment combining glucagon and GLP-1 can reduce appetite, according to research presented at a Society for Endocrinology's annual conference in Harrogate (March 2013). This study is reported to provide the "first in human" evidence of a combined therapy using these two hormones as the potential basis for future treatment of obesity and diabetes. Previous results in animal studies showed that a glucagon and GLP-1 combination might be effective in combating obesity and diabetes. As we've seen, glucagon works in opposition to insulin, preventing storage of glucose in fat deposits and the liver, and it raises blood sugar levels. GLP-1 stimulates the release of insulin to lower blood sugar and also acts within the brain to reduce appetite.

Scientists at the Toronto General Research Institute published a study in *Nature Medicine* online (2013) demonstrating that targeting glucagon action in the brain may be a new frontier for regulating diabetes. Glucagon is released when blood sugar levels fall too low and, as mentioned earlier, it functions in the liver to increase blood sugar levels. This increase, however, is temporary, and blood sugar levels return to normal. The contrary occurs in diabetes—glucagon's transient increase in blood sugar is impaired and levels remain elevated. Insulin is currently the most common means of regulating blood sugar balance in diabetics. Drugs that aim to increase glucagon action in the brain or block glucagon action in the liver could be the next superstars in the regulation of diabetic blood sugar levels.

Tips for a Glucagon Boost
Go, go, glucagon! It helps your fat be gone.

Foods and Habits
- **Nutrition:** Eat protein at every meal and keep blood sugars stable and regulated by avoiding excessive carbohydrates and combining protein, carbs, fat and fiber at each meal.
- **Exercise:** Yes! In studies involving both animal and human subjects exercising on a treadmill to exhaustion, glucagon was found to rise. Now, you certainly do not need to do this type of excessive activity. The Hormone Boost exercise prescription is just what you need.
- **Intermittent fasting:** Do the Hormone Boost fasting day.

Supplement Options
- Though there are no supplements to boost glucagon that I am aware of, protein powders are a simple way to stimulate glucagon on the go.

It's kind of fantastic that your body naturally *wants* to use sugar rather than protein as its primary fuel source. That's why glucagon is so imperative to your overall health. The tips in this book will help you navigate the good carb–bad carb maze, as well as give you the information you need to determine your best low-glycemic options.

But at the end of the day, hormones are about more than body fuel and energy levels. They're also about *how you feel*. That's where serotonin, dopamine and melatonin come in.

A HORMONE BOOST REAL-LIFE SUCCESS STORY

THE CLIENT: Franco S.

DETAILS: Male, 54

BODY COMPOSITION RESULTS (FROM SCALE AND BODY FAT/ MUSCLE MASS VIA BIO-IMPEDANCE TESTING)

MEASUREMENT	BEFORE	AFTER	TOTAL LOSS/GAIN
Weight (lb.)	194	185	(-) 9
Lean Body Mass (lb.)	156.4	156.0	(-) 0.4
Fat Mass (lb.)	37.6	29.0	(-) 8.6
Basal Metabolic Rate (calories/day)	2,212 calories	2,195 calories	(-) 12

They say 54 is the new 44—and this sure applies to Franco! He's a top hair stylist in Toronto and owner of one of the busiest salons in the city. He plays hockey and soccer with 30-year-olds—and they have trouble keeping up!

Franco didn't come with any specific complaints; he just wanted to "optimize what was right," making him a perfect example of the Hormone Boost philosophy. And the plan worked—he increased his energy, performance, mental focus, strength and vitality. *And he looked hot while doing it!*

Franco lost 8.6 pounds of fat while preserving his strength, and he hit his optimal body composition of 15.6 percent body fat at 54 years old. He sure is a star in my practice!

CHAPTER 7

BRAIN BOOST: HAPPY, MENTALLY SHARP AND CRAVING-FREE DOPAMINE, SEROTONIN AND MELATONIN

Be happy for this moment. This moment is your life.

OMAR KHAYYAM,

philosopher, poet and influential scientist of the Middle Ages

Because our bodies are hugely complex systems, it's sometimes easy to get lost in the details and forget how entwined our physiological and psychological states are. But they are, and this is where the three "hormone dwarves" come in; happy, driven and sleepy—as I like to call serotonin, dopamine and melatonin—have profound effects on the emotional texture of your day. Your mood, alertness, memory, self-esteem, sleeping patterns, cravings, eating habits and more rely on the proper regulation of this trusty trio.

The chemicals discussed in this chapter are both hormones and neurotransmitters (chemical messengers that work in the brain). They also affect concentration, weight and digestion, and they can cause adverse symptoms when they are out of balance. Stress, poor diet, neurotoxins, genetic predisposition, drugs (prescription and recreational), alcohol and caffeine can all change normal hormone levels, putting them out of the optimal range.

There are two types of neurotransmitters: inhibitory and excitatory. Inhibitory neurotransmitters, such as serotonin and dopamine, *calm* brain activity and balance mood. Excitatory neurotransmitters, such as dopamine (yes, dopamine does double duty) and norepinephrine, *stimulate* brain activity and motivation and improve focus.

Geek alert: Truth be told, I had a ton of fun combing through the latest research to compile the information in this chapter. Let's get to know these "three dwarves" a bit better.

Dopamine: The Pleasure Rush

If you are searching for stimulation or, as the song says, you feel you "can't get no satisfaction," you could probably use a good dose of dopamine. Dopamine is heavily involved in the brain's pleasure center. It's released in high amounts during gratifying activities— eating and having sex are probably the two that come to mind first, but dopamine is also released when we are in love, engaging in fun social interactions, giving, exercising and dancing, among other things.

As a brain chemical, dopamine influences pleasure, alertness, learning, creativity, attention and concentration. It also controls motor functions and muscle tension, which explains why a deficiency of this hormone is linked to Parkinson's disease and restless leg syndrome, as well as cognitive changes such as depression, low libido, attention disorders, memory loss and difficulties with problem solving.

While too little dopamine can leave us craving food, sex or stimulation, too much can cause addictive behaviors. For instance, Parkinson's patients taking medications to support dopamine levels have been shown to begin gambling when their medications are increased. Paranoia and suspicion may also arise from too much dopamine, although more of this hormone in the frontal area of the brain will relieve pain and boost pleasure. When it comes to dopamine, it's all about the right amount in the right place at the right time.

Dopamine for Weight Loss

Besides the many pleasures that dopamine brings, this phenomenal substance naturally suppresses appetite and aids weight loss. Antidepressant drugs such as bupropion (Wellbutrin or Zyban), which act on dopamine receptors in the brain, have been found to help with weight loss. A September 2002 study at Duke University Medical Center showed that weight loss occurred within just a few weeks and remained after a period of two years with bupropion use. Many of the study participants who took dopamine also reported feeling satisfied with smaller amounts of food.

Unfortunately, the body tends to work against itself when it comes to dopamine production. Way back in 1997, researchers at Princeton University found that dopamine *decreased* in rats when they lost weight on restricted eating programs. With this drop in weight, the rats' appetite increased and they began to eat more in an attempt to naturally restore dopamine levels. More recently, a study in *Psychoneuroendocrinology* (September 2014) found lower levels of dopamine associated with high carb intake. Luckily, the right diet and supplement prescription can optimize your brain level of dopamine and assist with appetite control.

Dopamine for Appetite Control

Mounting evidence shows that besides their ability to boost metabolism, hormones and neurotransmitters are involved in appetite control by acting on the hypothalamus gland, the part of the brain that governs our feelings of hunger and fullness. By collecting and processing information from the digestive system, the internal biological clock, fat cells, stress-controlling mechanisms and other sources within the body, the hypothalamus acts as the master switch that tells us when to eat more and when to stop.

In the midst of the current obesity epidemic, scientists are striving to understand both our struggle to gain control of our appetite and our tendency to overeat. They certainly have their work cut out for them!

COMPLEX FACTORS THAT INFLUENCE OUR NEED TO FEED

FACTORS THAT SPARK YOUR APPETITE	FACTORS THAT QUIET YOUR APPETITE
Sight and smell of food	Out of sight, out of mind
Overweight or obesity	Maintaining a lean body
Exposure to too many foods or tastes at once; standing in front of a buffet, fridge or cupboard (grazing is our downfall)	Limiting flavors and food variety in one sitting; avoiding buffets and grazing in front of the cupboard or fridge
Cold body temperature	Warm body temperature
Lack of sunlight or bright light exposure	A healthy dose of sunshine or bright light
Internal body clock: We tend to get hungry at similar times each day; appetite increases in the winter	Eating regularly throughout the day and *always* having breakfast
Alcohol consumption	Limiting consumption of alcohol to one glass of wine after your meal
Dehydration	Staying well hydrated
Jet lag, sleep deprivation and shift work	Sufficient, good-quality sleep
High intake of carbohydrates; lack of fiber and fats that help us feel full and satisfied	Consuming a mix of protein, carbohydrates, fiber and healthy fats at each meal and snack
Brain chemistry imbalance (low serotonin and dopamine); a compromised digestive system	Balanced brain chemistry (sufficient serotonin and dopamine); a healthy digestive system
High-fructose corn syrup (HFCS) and artificial sweeteners	Avoiding processed carbohydrates, artificial sweeteners, fructose and HFCS
Emotional causes: stress, anxiety, depression, loneliness, boredom	Managing stress and feeling satisfied (emotionally, sexually and otherwise)

While the environmental food cues outlined in the table on page 109 apply to all of us, it does appear that people who are obese may be more susceptible than their lean counterparts. According to a National Institutes of Health (NIH) study published in *Molecular Psychiatry* (October 2014), differences in brain chemistry can actually make eating more habitual and less rewarding. After examining 43 men and women with varying amounts of body fat, researchers at the NIH Clinical Center found that obese participants tended to have greater dopamine activity in the habit-forming region of the brain than lean participants, and less activity in the brain region that controls the sensation of reward. Those differences could potentially make obese people *more* drawn to overeat in response to food triggers, while simultaneously making food *less* rewarding. The researchers could not say whether obesity is a cause or an effect of this dopamine activity, since eating caused by unconscious habits rather than conscious choices could make it harder to achieve and maintain a healthy weight, especially when appetizing food cues are practically everywhere.

According to Dr. Kevin D. Hall, lead author and a senior investigator at the National Institute of Diabetes and Digestive and Kidney Diseases, cues like the smell of popcorn at the movies or an advertisement for a favorite food may have a stronger pull for an obese person—and a stronger reaction from their brain chemistry—than for a lean person exposed to the same trigger.

So it now seems that even our *amount* of body fat influences how we process information about food. However, keeping dopamine levels high could help mitigate this increased desire to eat, since eating and dopaminergic signaling are closely related. Food rewards and food reward–associated stimuli both elevate dopamine levels in crucial components of the brain's reward circuits. In fact, food might be the most important natural stimulator of that reward system. So overeating might actually be your brain's way of attempting to compensate for low dopamine activity. It doesn't matter if the suppressed levels of dopamine are the result of genetics or the fallout of fewer dopamine rushes after, say, the cessation of smoking or less overindulgence with large amounts of highly addictive foods. In either case, leveling off dopamine levels—to maintain the brain's influence on the drive *not* to eat—is crucial to preventing weight gain.

The story of the happy and craving-free brain may start with dopamine, but it certainly doesn't stop there. Serotonin is next on your list for a brain boost.

The Sweet Comfort of Serotonin

Though serotonin is typically recognized as a brain chemical, the majority of this neurotransmitter is produced in our digestive tract. Serotonin exerts a powerful influence over mood, emotions, memory, cravings (especially for carbohydrates), self-esteem, pain tolerance, sleep habits, appetite, digestion and body temperature regulation. Wow! When we're depressed or down, we naturally crave sugars and starches to stimulate the production of serotonin. Also, when we're cold or surrounded by darkness, serotonin levels drop—which explains that dreaded winter weight gain.

Serotonin is often thought of as our "happy hormone," especially because its production increases when we're exposed to natural sunlight and when we focus on one thing rather than multitask. Serotonin production is also closely linked to the availability of vitamin B_6 and the amino acid tryptophan (the precursor to serotonin). So, if our diet lacks sufficient protein or vitamins, we run a greater risk of serotonin deficiency. We may experience a dip in serotonin in relation to physiological causes, dieting, digestive disorders and also stress, since high levels of the stress hormone cortisol rob us of serotonin.

Serotonin and Appetite Regulation

Serotonin has also been implicated in controlling how much food we eat during a sitting and how often we feel the need to eat. The mechanism for this control lies within the serotonin receptors in our central nervous system. These receptors are sensitive to circulating levels of tryptophan, macronutrients and cholecystokinin (CCK), which controls our sensation of fullness.

Serotonin receptors in the hypothalamus also *inhibit* neuropeptide Y (NPY), a potent stress hormone that's also a stimulator of hunger and food intake. Serotonin is a part of an integrated network for short-acting appetite control, while leptin is a hormonal indicator of long-term fat and energy reserves. In other words, serotonin satisfies our appetite in the here and now and leptin is the long-term driving force that keeps it in check. Both work by adjusting NPY activity.

What's more, according to research connecting serotonin with carbohydrate craving, obesity and depression from the Massachusetts Institute of Technology (November 1995), serotonin-releasing brain neurons are unique in that *the amount of serotonin they release is dependent on food intake.* So, carbohydrate consumption increases serotonin release; protein intake does not. Researchers found evidence to support what many of us already know—many patients *learn* to overeat carbohydrates, particularly snack foods rich in carbohydrates and fats, because they make them feel better.

The prevalent tendency to use certain carb-rich foods as though they were drugs (i.e., mood-altering substances) is a frequent cause of weight gain. It is also an underlying factor in patients who gain fat when exposed to stress, in women with premenstrual syndrome, in patients with "winter depression" and in those attempting to give up smoking. Regardless of the cause of your stress, it is that stress that causes you to abandon your diet and reach for the comforts in the cupboard.

Studies from way back have shown how serotonin rises in the bloodstream after we eat a carb-rich meal, as opposed to a meal high in fat and protein. But keep this in mind: The increase in serotonin is a desired effect after our evening meal. Not only does it help body composition and appetite control, it also helps enhance sleep. This goes against the advice of weight-loss and bodybuilding gurus who have advocated, for years and years, eating carbs in the morning, with the suggestion that there is a greater chance to burn them off throughout the day.

Fitness and training guru Charles Poliquin has promoted eating carbs in the evening since 1982, as stated in his article "The Case for Eating Your Carbohydrates at Night—Revised." He sometimes quotes a later reference as one source of support: A 1997 study published in the *Journal of Nutrition* that showed how eating the vast majority of carbs (70 percent of your daily intake) in the evening as part of a moderate diet appears to cause more fat loss, even though less total body weight is lost. Results suggested that less muscle is lost when carbs are consumed in the evening. A more recent study (2014) supports eating carbohydrates mostly at dinner—and protein mostly at lunch—within a low-calorie balanced diet, because this approach has a higher effect on fat-burning. The reverse—eating carbohydrates mostly at lunch and protein mostly at dinner—turns out to have a damaging impact on blood sugar control.

So what does this mean for you? Eat a meal rich in protein and good fat first thing in the morning (meal 1), meals rich in carbs sourced from green vegetables, protein and fat during the day (meals 2 and 3—with fruit as a carb source in one of these meals) and a meal that includes a starchy carb selection with protein and fat in the evening (meal 4). This is the Hormone Boost's energy, strength and weight-loss enhancing plan.

Serotonin and Brown Fat

Researchers from McMaster University have identified an important hormone that shows up in high levels in obese people; this hormone contributes to obesity and diabetes by impeding brown fat activity. Brown fat is located around the collarbone, functions as the body's furnace to burn calories and keeps the body warm. Obese people have less of it, and its activity decreases with age. Until now, researchers haven't understood why.

It turns out that there are two types of serotonin. Most people are familiar with the first type, which functions in the brain or central nervous system and affects mood and appetite. But this makes up *only* 5 percent of the body's serotonin. (Really—I was shocked when I first read this too!) The lesser-known peripheral serotonin circulates in the blood and makes up the other 95 percent of the body's serotonin. It turns out that this kind of serotonin reduces brown fat activity—"dials down" the body's metabolic furnace—which is not the ideal situation for good health. The study, published in *Nature Medicine* (2014), is the first to show that blocking the production of peripheral serotonin makes brown fat more active.

Dr. Gregory Steinberg, the paper's co-author and professor of medicine at the Michael G. DeGroote School of Medicine, is also codirector of MAC-Obesity, the Metabolism and Childhood Obesity Research Program at McMaster. His research suggests that the culprit responsible for elevated levels of peripheral serotonin may be environmental—the availability of high-fat foods, which comprise such a large part of the Western diet. Too much of even a good thing like serotonin can be harmful and can lead to diabetes, fatty liver and obesity.

Serotonin: The Missing Link

Although essential marine omega-3 fatty acids and vitamin D have been shown to improve cognitive function and behavior in the context of certain brain disorders, the underlying mechanism has been unclear. A paper in the *FASEB Journal* (February 2015) offers a potential explanation: Serotonin might be the missing link that explains how and why vitamin D and marine omega-3 fatty acids can alleviate symptoms associated with a broad array of disorders.

This group of researchers has looked into previous studies on how vitamin D regulates the conversion of tryptophan into serotonin, exploring how this conversion might influence the development of autism, particularly in children with poor vitamin D status. Their work considers the relevance of these nutrients for neuropsychiatric illness. We know that serotonin affects a wide range of cognitive functions and behaviors, including mood, social behavior and impulsive behavior. It even plays a role in social decision-making by keeping aggressive responses or impulsive behaviors in check. Many clinical disorders, such as autism spectrum disorder, attention deficit hyperactivity disorder (ADHD), bipolar disorder, schizophrenia, anxiety and depression, have low brain serotonin in common.

Eicosapentaenoic acid (EPA) increases serotonin release from presynaptic neurons by reducing the inflammatory signals in the brain that can inhibit serotonin release. This explains how inflammation may negatively impact serotonin in the brain. EPA, however, is not the only omega-3 that plays a role in the serotonin pathway. Docosahexaenoic acid (DHA) also influences the action of various serotonin receptors; it makes them more accessible to serotonin by increasing cell membrane fluidity in neurons. The takeaway? Optimize your intake of vitamin D, EPA and DHA. They help to optimize brain serotonin status and function.

Marvelous Melatonin: Great Sleep, Strong Muscles and a Lean Body

Another hormone closely related to serotonin (it is also produced from tryptophan) is melatonin. And it can be your secret weapon. Melatonin is released from the pineal gland and regulates your natural 24-hour body clock. Melatonin normally increases after darkness falls, making us feel drowsy. Acting as a hormone, melatonin influences nervous system function as well as the endocrine and immune systems. Its production typically peaks between 1 and 3 a.m., while you are asleep in the dark. Exposure to even small amounts of light (from, say, your digital alarm clock) or to electromagnetic radiation (from alarm clocks, TVs, heating pads or electric blankets) disrupts this process. Your melatonin production can also be compromised if you regularly take aspirin or ibuprofen, consume caffeinated products, drink alcohol or smoke.

Because melatonin is a derivative of serotonin, its production is also dependent on adequate protein in your diet; protein provides tryptophan, the amino acid building block of both melatonin and serotonin. Melatonin naturally tends to decline with aging and menopause, which makes supplementation a helpful natural option for people over 45 and for those who experience sleep problems.

Melatonin's Nighttime Magic

Melatonin is a powerful antioxidant that maintains youthfulness, improves sleep, perks up libido and boosts energy and resistance to infections. It affects your ability to fall asleep, stay asleep and experience quality sleep. It also indirectly influences your body composition through its relationship with growth hormone, which you will remember from Chapter 4.

Melatonin essentially helps turn on the body's nighttime repair processes by allowing for a slight but essential dip in body temperature. Once your body has cooled sufficiently, growth hormone is released and begins to work its magic, repairing and rebuilding bone, skin and muscle cells as you sleep. As an added bonus, melatonin decreases cortisol and protects us from the harmful effects of stress. Thanks to its dual effects on growth hormone and cortisol, melatonin helps our metabolic rate by preserving muscle tissue.

The Link between Melatonin and Serotonin

When melatonin goes up, serotonin goes down. The most common example of this is that melatonin levels rise in the winter when we have less sunlight exposure. The correlative drop in serotonin is thought to be one of the main causes of seasonal depression, also known as seasonal affective disorder (SAD). Increased carbohydrate cravings and weight gain are common symptoms of SAD. Eating more carbs in turn causes the body to step up its production of serotonin. This technique can be an effective way to keep negative moods at bay, as long as it is used in moderation. This is the reason why I recommend avoiding starchy carb–free diets, especially in the winter. Unfortunately, we tend to overeat comfort foods such as chips, cookies and candy, which pump up serotonin and leave us feeling fat, fuzzy and even more depressed.

A New Relationship between Melatonin and Dopamine

In 2012 a group of Spanish researchers discovered a new relationship between dopamine and melatonin, according to *PLOS Biology*. We know that dopamine acts in the pineal gland, which dictates the circadian rhythm in humans—that series of biological processes that enables brain activity to adapt to the time of day (that is, to light and dark cycles). Another hormone, norepinephrine, is involved in promoting this synthesis and the release of melatonin in the pineal gland.

When dopamine interacts with its

Good News for a Wine-Based NightCap?

The grapes used to make some of the most popular red wines contain high levels of melatonin, according to scientists from the University of Milan (*Journal of the Science of Food and Agriculture*, June 2006). This could be the reason that so many of us reach for a glass in the evening to "wind down" after a hard day's slog.

For a long time, melatonin was thought to be produced exclusively by mammals, but it has recently been discovered in plants and now in wine—in the Nebbiolo, Merlot, Cabernet Sauvignon, Sangiovese and Croatina grape varieties. But don't rush to the wine store just yet. Dr. Richard Wurtman of the Brain and Cognitive Science Department at the Massachusetts Institute of Technology is unconvinced; he believes that further research is needed to determine whether the compounds discovered are melatonin or something very similar.

receptors, it inhibits the effects of norepinephrine, which means a decrease in the production and release of melatonin. Interestingly, researchers found that these dopamine receptors appear in the pineal gland only toward the end of the night, as the dark period closes. The researchers' conclusion is that these receptors are an effective mechanism to stop melatonin production and wake up the brain when the day begins.

Their results demonstrate a mechanism in which dopamine, normally increased at times of stimulation, can directly inhibit the production and release of melatonin that induces drowsiness and prepares the body for sleep. This makes sense, since we want melatonin levels to drop in the morning and dopamine levels to rise—both processes need to happen for our brains to wake up. The discovery could be extremely useful when designing new treatments to help mitigate circadian rhythm disturbances, such as those related to jet lag, shift work and sleep disorders in general, which, according to the World Health Organization, affect 40 percent of the world's population.

Melatonin and Sleep Efficiency

If you're looking for more evidence that melatonin improves sleep quality, consider this: Researchers from the divisions of sleep medicine at Brigham and Women's Hospital and Harvard Medical School have found that melatonin taken orally during nontypical sleep times (i.e., during the day) significantly improves our ability to sleep (*Sleep*, May 2006). This is great news for night-shift workers, jet-lagged travelers and sufferers from advanced and delayed sleep phase syndrome.

Participants ingested either a placebo, 0.3 mg of pharmaceutical-grade melatonin or 5 mg of pharmaceutical-grade melatonin. Sleep efficiency during the 6-hour-and-40-minute episodes was significantly higher in the groups that took melatonin *during times when the body was not producing melatonin*. At those times, participants taking 5.0 mg of melatonin had a sleep efficiency of 83 percent, and those taking 0.3 mg of melatonin had a sleep efficiency of 84 percent. This was significantly better than the placebo group, who had a sleep efficiency of 77 percent.

The results definitively showed that the use of melatonin as a sleep aid was beneficial when the body wasn't already releasing its own supply of melatonin. They leave little doubt about melatonin's effectiveness in alleviating sleep disturbances when attempting to sleep at the wrong time of day. Interestingly, melatonin did not help these young adults sleep at night, when their body was already producing melatonin.

Many of my patients and Hormone Diet boot-campers have heard me prescribe Clear Balance—Stress Support Formula with melatonin for shift workers. I used to prescribe melatonin as part of this sleep treatment protocol only on the nights when the shift workers slept like the rest of us. Based on this study's results, I now suggest 3 mg of Clear ZZZ's—Melatonin and two capsules of Clear Balance at bedtime, regardless of when that is, and one capsule of Clear Balance upon rising, to balance cortisol while awake.

Melatonin for Your Circadian Clock

My husband is an outdoors fanatic: he loves being at the cottage and he loves camping. If he had his way, he would be pleased as punch to chop wood and have a bonfire going at all times. And it seems that all this camping activity is good not just for his soul but also for his sleep. Have you ever noticed how, when you're exposed to natural sunlight, your internal clock becomes perfectly synchronized to the solar day? I bet you didn't realize this shift can happen in less than a week.

The reason for this is explained in a *Current Biology* study (August 2013), which showed that spending just one week exposed only to natural light while camping in the Rocky Mountains was enough to sync the circadian clocks of eight people. The synchronization happened regardless of whether the participants were early birds or night owls in their normal lives.

It's impossible not to experience some kind of fallout with our circadian clocks in this fast-paced 24-hour, always-connected world. Part of the departure from our natural synchronized timing may initially have been the result of electric lighting, which became widely available in the 1930s. Electric lighting affects our internal clocks and lets *us* decide when to tell our bodies to prepare for sleep and when to prepare for waking. The ability to flip a switch and flood a room with light allows us to be exposed to light much later into the night than would be naturally possible. What's more, even when we are exposed to electric lights during daylight hours, the intensity of indoor lighting is much less than that of sunlight, and the color of electric light also differs from natural light, which changes shades throughout the day.

Researchers had a unique approach to testing the effect of electric light versus natural light—they gave participants wrist monitors that recorded the intensity of the light they were exposed to, the timing of that light, and their activity. This information then allowed the researchers to map out their sleeping patterns. In the first week of the study, participants went about their regular lives at home and work. At week's end, their melatonin levels were measured. The same metrics were recorded during and after a second week, when the eight participants went camping in Colorado's Eagles Nest Wilderness. During the week, the campers were exposed only to sunlight and the glow of a campfire. Flashlights and personal electronic devices were not allowed.

After the camping trip—wherein the subjects were exposed to *four times* the intensity of light in their normal lives—participants' biological nighttime began near sunset and ended at sunrise. They also woke up just after their biological night had ended. During their normal lives, complete with exposure to electric light, the participants' biological nighttime started roughly *two hours later.* They also woke up before their biological night had ended.

Living in the modern world gives us the opportunity for individualization; we can choose to be early birds or night owls (or, if we're unlucky, our responsibilities make that choice for us). While some of us are naturally morning types and others like to stay up later, natural light/dark cycles provide a strong signal that dramatically reduces the differences we see among people.

That's how strong a single stint of seven days' exposure to natural light was, and it offers potential solutions for those of us who struggle with sleep. People who naturally drift toward staying up late may also find that it's more difficult to feel alert in the morning. We now know that in those instances, melatonin levels could indicate that they're still in their biological nighttime—regardless of whether they're physically at work or in school.

There is an answer, and it's simple—combat the drift toward later nights with exposure to more sunlight in the morning and midday. Dimming your lights at night (a habit I've had for years, even when visiting friends at their homes) and forgoing late-night TV helps (though using the sleep function to ensure the TV turns off makes me less opposed to vegging out to the TV than I am to computer use, which definitely stimulates more brain activity). Cutting out late-night screen time with laptops and other personal electronic devices is vital to help your internal clock stay more closely attuned with the sun. Because sleep is so integral to hormonal harmony, getting the best sleep you can is at the top of the priority list for the Hormone Boost.

Melatonin for Control of Weight Gain

According to a study published in the *Journal of Pineal Research* (2010) by University of Granada researchers, melatonin can help control weight gain in animals, even without reducing food intake. Melatonin also reduces triglycerides and increases HDL (good) cholesterol while reducing LDL (bad) cholesterol.

Interestingly, melatonin is found in small quantities in some fruits and vegetables—mustard, goji berries, almonds, sunflower seeds, cardamom, fennel, coriander and cherries all have small amounts. Bringing these foods into your diet could help manage weight gain and prevent the heart diseases associated with obesity as well as triglyceride and cholesterol imbalances. If this finding is confirmed in humans, the administration of melatonin and intake of foods containing melatonin might be a useful tool to fight obesity and its inherent risks.

Melatonin consumption appears to help control weight gain because it stimulates the appearance of beige fat, a type of fat cell that burns calories instead of storing them. White adipose tissue stores calories, leading to weight gain, whereas beige fat (also known as "good" or "thinning" fat) helps regulate body weight control. And that's a serious metabolic benefit.

Melatonin for Bone Strength

McGill University researchers have shown that melatonin supplements may make bones stronger in old rats, suggesting a possible avenue for the prevention of osteoporosis. Bones are built up by certain cells, known as osteoblasts, during the day and broken down by others, known as osteoclasts, at night.

Giving elderly rats melatonin supplements to regulate their circadian rhythms seems to make their bones denser, less brittle and more flexible. The next step is to explore whether melatonin supplements prevent bone breakdown or can actually repair damage. The latter seems possible, and that would be great news indeed.

Research on bones and melatonin is trending now, in fact. A study completed across the pond, by researchers at the University of Madrid (*Rejuvenation Research*, 2014), is based on a very interesting comparison of 22-month-old rats and 60-year-old humans (when it comes to bone density, it seems they are equivalent). Researchers gave 20 rats melatonin supplements diluted in water for ten weeks (the equivalent of six human years). The femurs taken from the elderly rats that had received the melatonin supplements were then compared with those of a control group that had not received the supplements, using a series of tests to measure bone density and strength.

A significant increase in both bone volume and density occurred among the rats that had received melatonin supplements. As a result, the bones broke less readily, which suggests that melatonin may prove a useful tool in combating osteoporosis.

Tips for a Boost of Dopamine, Serotonin and Melatonin

A serotonin, dopamine and melatonin boost can go a long way to ensuring that your days are happy, your mind is calm, your sleep is restful and your body is relaxed. Who would say no to that?

Foods and Habits That Increase Dopamine

- **Nutrition:** Make an effort to consume proteins (meat, milk products, fish, beans, nuts, soy products), but especially turkey, which is high in phenylalanine, the building block of dopamine. Phenylalanine is found in most protein-rich foods, so eat them when you want to feel sharper. Coffee may also stimulate dopamine release.
- **Eat breakfast:** A new study has found that eating breakfast—especially one that includes foods rich in protein (see above)—increases dopamine levels, which can help reduce food cravings and overeating later in the day. A 2012 University of Missouri study, published in *Nutrition Journal,* showed that people who eat breakfast experience a dramatic decline in sweet food cravings. Breakfasts that are high in protein also reduce cravings for savory—or high-fat—foods. If breakfast is skipped, however, these cravings continue to rise throughout the day. Give yourself the best start to your day with a fat- and protein-rich breakfast. And don't forget

your sources of tyrosine to increase the production of dopamine: almonds, avocados, bananas, dairy products, lima beans, pumpkin seeds and sesame seeds.

- **Exercise:** As you may have noticed by now, exercise is an integral part of producing the hormones you need to be your best self. For dopamine increases specifically, try changing up your workouts often—this can be as simple as choosing a different running or walking route. More changes in your workout boost dopamine.
- **Sex:** Sex provides a nice dose of dopamine, which increases steadily to the point of orgasm and then declines. Apparently the dopamine pathways in the brain involved in stimulating desire for both sex and food are shut down by the hormones released immediately after we have an orgasm. Can you imagine better news for appetite and craving control?
- **Massage:** At least once a month. Your body, mind and soul will thank you.

Supplement Options to Increase Dopamine

- **Clear Energy – Dopamine Support Formula:** Revitalize your brain, energy and metabolism with this herbal combination that specifically provides a wonderful dose of dopamine. I blend L-tyrosine, D-phenylalanine and rhodiola to boost metabolic power and brain energy. Take two to three pills upon rising, before breakfast.
- **L-tyrosine:** The amino acid tyrosine is a building block of dopamine, so supplements can definitely perk up production of this mood-influencing hormone. Take 500 to 1,000 mg upon rising, away from food. Another dose may be added later in the day, but because tyrosine is a stimulating supplement, it should not be taken after 3 p.m., and *it should be completely avoided by anyone with high blood pressure.* This product should be taken for at least four to six weeks to reach

full effectiveness. Tyrosine is the best choice if low thyroid hormone or underactive thyroid is also suspected.

- **D- or DL-phenylalanine:** Like tyrosine, phenylalanine is a building block of dopamine. A study published in one German psychiatry journal showed that phenylalanine was as effective as certain antidepressant drugs. Take 500 to 1,000 mg daily, away from food, before 3 p.m. As with tyrosine, phenylalanine must be taken for at least four to six weeks for full effectiveness. *DL-phenylalanine may be the better choice if you also have body aches and pains.*

- **Rhodiola:** Rhodiola can enhance learning capacity and memory and may also be useful for treating fatigue, stress and depression. Research suggests rhodiola may enhance mood regulation and fight depression by stimulating the activity of serotonin and dopamine. Take 200 to 400 mg daily in the morning, away from food, for a minimum of one month.

- **Chasteberry (vitex):** Chasteberry has been shown to increase both dopamine and progesterone, making it an excellent choice for women who experience symptoms of depression in conjunction with PMS or irregular menstrual cycles. Take 200 mg of a 10:1 extract each morning before breakfast for one to six months.

Foods and Habits That Increase Serotonin

- **Nutrition:** Eating carbohydrates will boost your serotonin, so choose slow-release complex carbs, including whole-grain breads, brown rice and pasta, to keep you sustained, energized and balanced. Simple carbs such as white bread and pastries will provide only a momentary boost followed by a crash—plus they pack on the fat, so avoid them. The best food sources of serotonin-boosting tryptophan are brown rice, cottage cheese, meat, peanuts and sesame seeds. Chia seeds contain tryptophan too.

- **Slow it down:** Meditating or focusing your mind on one thing is an important part of making the most of your serotonin levels. Effective multitasking is a myth, so avoid trying to take on more than one task at a time!
- **Sun exposure:** A moderate dose of sunshine is great for serotonin levels and vitamin D.
- **Temperature:** Stay warm. Evidently serotonin neurons can be activated by warm temperatures externally (via the skin) and internally. There is merit to the depression "a warm, fuzzy feeling." And if you needed justification to buy a hot tub, *boom!*—you just found it.
- **Exercise:** Yes! High-intensity exercise (where you break a nice sweat—with sprinting, interval cardio or a Hormone Boost strength-training session) is often best. You must, however, do it every 48 hours (and no further apart) to gain mood- and serotonin-enhancing effects. Add music to your workouts too. It's proven to raise serotonin and dopamine and improve your performance.
- **Massage:** Once or twice a month.

Supplement Options to Boost Serotonin
- **Clear Mood – Serotonin Support Formula:** This effective formula contains all the ingredients needed to increase your serotonin for better mood, appetite, sleep, digestion, memory and pain relief. I have included vitamins B_6, B_{12}, 5-HTP, St. John's wort and folic acid. Take two capsules before bed and one capsule in the morning. If they make you feel nauseated when taken on an empty stomach in the morning, try them with your protein smoothie or at bedtime instead. This product must be taken consistently for four to six weeks to reach full effectiveness.
- **5-HTP:** A derivative of tryptophan and one step closer to becoming serotonin, 5-hydroxytryptophan (5-HTP) has

been found to be more effective than tryptophan for treating sleeplessness, depression, anxiety and fibromyalgia. Take 50 to 400 mg daily, in divided doses throughout the day or before bed. This product should be taken for at least four to six weeks to reach full effectiveness.

- **Vitamin B$_6$:** Vitamin B$_6$ supports the production and function of serotonin in the brain. Take 50 to 100 mg before bed.
- **Rhodiola:** Rhodiola may enhance learning capacity, memory and mood regulation. It may also help fight depression by stimulating the activity of serotonin and dopamine. Take 200 to 400 mg daily, preferably in the morning.
- **St. John's wort:** This herb has proven effective for easing mild to moderate depression. It appears to work as a natural SSRI by preventing the breakdown of serotonin in the brain. It takes at least four to six weeks to reach full effectiveness. Recommended dosage is 900 mg daily, away from food.
- **Inositol:** Naturally present in many foods, inositol improves the activity of serotonin in the brain. As a supplement, it is an excellent choice for alleviating anxiety and depression and supporting nervous system health. I use it in powdered form and add it to my daily smoothie. Take 4 to 12 g daily. When mixed with magnesium, inositol is very effective for calming the nervous system.

Foods and Habits That Increase Melatonin

- **Nutrition:** Consume protein, particularly sources that contain the tryptophan needed to make melatonin, such as pumpkin seeds, chia seeds and walnuts. Natural cherry juice has also been shown to increase melatonin.
- **Sleep:** Total darkness and coolness are your best bet for deep and effective sleep. Follow the habits for healthy sleep outlined in the Hormone Boost's simple steps in Chapter 8.

- **Light:** Expose yourself to bright light immediately upon rising and throughout the day; keep the lights dim after dinner and avoid the temptation of screen time! Bonus points if you can get your natural circadian rhythms back on track.

Supplement Options to Boost Melatonin

- **Melatonin:** Take 0.5 to 10 mg daily at bedtime to aid sleep. It is most effective when taken in lozenge or spray form. Here's a tip: Feeling groggy in the morning usually means you took your melatonin supplement too late in the evening or in too high a dose for your needs.

You can boost your moods, control your appetite and even regulate your body clock by attending to your dopamine, serotonin and melatonin through the suggestions in this chapter. As you'll see in the next section, there are three simple principles you can follow to align everything you've read so far with the Hormone Boost your body needs.

A HORMONE BOOST REAL-LIFE SUCCESS STORY

THE CLIENT: Emily B.

DETAILS: Female, 24

BODY COMPOSITION RESULTS (FROM SCALE AND BODY FAT/ MUSCLE MASS VIA BIO-IMPEDANCE TESTING)

MEASUREMENT	BEFORE	AFTER	TOTAL LOSS/GAIN
Weight (lb.)	73	100	(+) 27
Lean Body Mass (lb.)	53.7	72.1	(+) 18.4
Fat Mass (lb.)	19.3	27.9	(+) 8.6
Basal Metabolic Rate (calories/day)	758 calories	1,101 calories	(+) 343

There's one patient I always make sure to hug before she leaves the office: Emily. I am so proud of her and her transformation—an incredible example of a Hormone Boost of *strength*. In a period of just five months she restored her lean body mass (muscle and bone) and gained enough weight to free her from the health risks of being underweight and undernourished.

Emily has struggled with digestive problems (heartburn, bloating and spasms, which we are still working on today), but her energy, vitality, sleep, mental functions and strength are all much improved. Emily's case demonstrates that a hormone boost isn't always about losing weight; it's about achieving hormonal health and all the benefits that come with it.

She's so committed, and every time I see her working out with Anthony, our strength-trailing report, she scores major admiration points in my book.

PART TWO

GET PREPPED

If you want to achieve excellence, you can get there today.
As of this second, quit doing less-than-excellent work.

THOMAS J. WATSON,
American businessman, former chairman and CEO of IBM

CHAPTER 8

THREE-STEP HOME PREP

*I told my mother-in-law that my house was her house,
and she said, "Get the hell off my property."*

JOAN RIVERS

Okay, enough talk already. Now that we've learned all about the fat-loss six and how these hard-working hormones can be your secret weapons in the quest for better overall health, it's time to put theory into practice. In this chapter, I will guide you through a step-by-step preparation designed to get you ready for your Hormone Boost. A new season, the transition to fall, New Year's—even any given Monday—can be the perfect time to start a new health regimen. The recommendations presented here will help you implement new behaviors—and, even more importantly, stick with them. Ready?

It All Starts at Home

Healthy habits aren't all about your body. I fully woke up to the link between environment and well-being two years ago, when my husband and I downsized from our house to a condo. Amid the chaos of half-unpacked boxes, I realized just how important an uncluttered and organized living space is. Our habits suffered because groceries were sparse, pots were MIA, dishes were still packed and our supplements were out of sight. We tripped into bed at night over piles of clothes and folded linens. And during the day, we felt beyond worn out from the constant mental chatter of our to-do lists, and simply because we were unsettled.

No wonder. Piles and piles of laundry and endless to-dos are exhausting. They also mess with your hormones and your health (mental and physical). In the introduction, I wrote about the "TurnTash Method"—my silly spin on the popular KonMari Method, which offers a way to declutter your life and bring joy. Embracing this level of organization will make more time for *you*, and enable you to live the Hormone Boost lifestyle. Consider the following benefits.

- **You will be more successful and lose more weight.** Organization heightens your ability to be mindful about what you put into your body. My own experience tells me that success begins with thoughts or ideas, takes shape with planning, organization and preparation, and comes to fruition with motivation and commitment to follow through.
- **You will sleep better.** I've said it before and I will say it again: clutter is a state of mind. The one room in your whole house that *must* be free of clutter is your bedroom. Yet, as one of my patients stated the other day, the bedroom is all too often the most cluttered room in the house. (Who isn't guilty of stashing stuff there before a party or family dinner?) In August 2015, I organized my mother's bedroom (actually, her whole house). I cleared piles of books, horse bridles, purses, papers and all other forms of clutter from her floor space. I organized her drawers, purged old clothes, organized her closet—and guess what? She started sleeping better. Her mind was more at peace in a clean, clear and uncluttered sleeping space. Less mess equals less stress, which naturally results in better sleep. But keeping your bedroom neat may

benefit your slumber in other ways too. According to a National Sleep Foundation poll on bedroom habits (sleepfoundation.org), people who make their beds every morning are 19 percent more likely to report regularly getting a good night's rest, and 75 percent of people said they got a better night's sleep when their sheets were fresh and clean, because they were more comfortable. A word of warning: Chaos throughout your day can lead you to bring last-minute tasks—such as paying bills and writing emails—into your bedroom. And that can cause you to stay up longer and get on the computer (a definite no-no at night), making it more difficult to nod off. So don't leave all the organizing until the end of the day!

- **You will make Hormone Boost–friendly food choices.** Incredibly, a study from *Psychological Science* (December 2012) found that people who worked in a neat space for 10 minutes were twice as likely to choose an apple over a chocolate bar than those who worked in a messy office for the same amount of time. Clutter at work or home is stressful for the brain, which makes you more likely to resort (consciously or unconsciously) to coping mechanisms such as choosing comfort foods or overeating. Plus, kitchen decluttering, "detoxing" of hormone disruptors (outlined later in this chapter) and planning the organization of foods and meals (stocking up on nutritious foods; preparing protein-rich meal-on-the-go options and smoothies; prepping fruits and vegetables) will only help to ensure that you make Hormone Boost eating your reality.
- **You will exercise more.** I love scanning my monthly planner and seeing workouts recorded on most days of the week. Yup, I schedule my workouts—and it seems this is what's required to make us more successful, according to a report in the *Journal of Obesity* (2011). This simple habit will

motivate you to go to your workouts and keep on going. Try to record as much information as you can about duration, weights, sets, reps, etc.

- **You will have more room for the new.** My hubby thinks I have a bit of OCD. Before every vacation, I have to tidy our home, do all the laundry, put it all away and *then* pack. And when I write, I have to clean every room—especially the area where I am working. Clutter distracts me. (So do email pop-ups; I turn them off and check my email only every hour or so.) It seems my need to be clean and tidy isn't unique. Research confirms that clutter affects our ability to focus, because looking at too many things at once overloads our visual cortex, which impacts our brain's ability to process information (*Journal of Neuroscience*, January 2011). Being more productive and efficient is also a natural by-product of an orderly home or workspace—less time is wasted searching for things! Imagine how much more productive and creative you might be with a bit more time.

- **You will be in a better mood, feel happier and have stronger relationships**. Women who described their homes as "cluttered" or full of "unfinished projects" were more depressed and fatigued and had higher levels of the stress hormone cortisol than women who felt their homes were "restful" and "restorative," according to a study in *Personality and Social Psychology Bulletin* (2010). It's no wonder: Coming home to piles of things or a huge to-do list may prevent the natural decline in stress and cortisol that should occur over the course of the day. Trying to relax in clutter or untidiness only furthers stress and, if you live with a partner, can lead to tension, conflict and wasted time. ("Honey, have you seen my . . .") Last, when it comes to other relationships, a messy house may also prevent you from inviting people over. So be a good girl or boy—go clean your room!

Convinced now? I certainly hope so. It's obvious that paying attention to your surroundings pays off—big time—when it comes to your health. Various chemicals and hormone disruptors are lurking in your environment that can interfere with your boost. So our first step is to get rid of those nasty things, and the logical place to start is—no surprise—the kitchen.

Step 1: The Kitchen Boost

When it comes to starting any new personal health regimen, the kitchen is surely target number one. So many bad habits are formed—and fed—in this important spot in your home. Before you start your Hormone Boost, it's vital that you spend a bit of time in the kitchen, making sure there's nothing standing in the way of your success. After all, lurking in your kitchen are foods that can derail you in a big way. Let's start with a list of foods you should never eat; in fact, I recommend that you remove them from your kitchen immediately to prevent further hormonal disruption.

- Products containing artificial sweeteners (aspartame, sucralose, etc.)
- Products containing high-fructose corn syrup
- Vegetable oil, shortening, margarine, cottonseed oil; anything containing partially hydrogenated oils; products containing trans fats
- Processed and packaged foods that contain lots of preservatives, loads of sodium and few nutrients (e.g., prepared pasta or rice side dishes)

Once you've got a handle on your cupboards and fridge, the next step of your kitchen boost is to get rid of your plastic food-storage containers and replace them with glass. Use paper wraps instead of plastic whenever possible; if you do use plastic wraps, make sure that those you put in contact with food do not contain phthalates (chemical compounds that act like harmful estrogens in the body and are known to increase the risk of breast cancer, prostate cancer, low testosterone in men, and smaller penis size in babies when the mother is exposed). If you're not sure, ask the manufacturer. And *never* microwave food in plastic containers or polystyrene foam, which may leach harmful compounds. Potentially harmful or cancer-causing estrogen-like chemicals in plastic, called dioxins, can seep into your foods and drinks, especially when heated or frozen. Always choose metal, glass or wood instead of plastic for storing, reheating and serving foods. The glass jars that some foods come in, such as pickles or olives, can be reused as storage for other foods—at no extra cost to you.

What about soft plastic water bottles? We've all heard about the potential dangers of BPA and other plastic chemicals, and the reports are accurate. Higher amounts of these chemicals are linked to more abdominal fat and changes in the brain and endocrine system. Avoid these as much as you can, and *never* drink your water from your plastic water bottle if it has been heated or frozen in your car. Do not refill disposable bottles. When you need to purchase water or juice products, try to buy those that come in glass bottles, or treat yourself to a beautiful and practical reusable bottle; glass, stainless steel and bamboo options are all available, and some are real works of art. You may also want to consider a reverse-osmosis water system for your kitchen tap. It is much less expensive than buying a unit for the whole house. I have one installed at my clinic, cottage and home—I highly recommend it as a means of removing toxins, heavy metals, bacteria and other impurities from your drinking water. You may want to check out a new source of hydration recently released by a company based in Toronto, called GP8 Oxygen Water. This amazing water, sold in BPA-free bottles, uses a unique electrolysis technology to create a product with four times more soluble oxygen. It is also reverse-osmosis water and pH (alkaline) optimized.

When it comes to food preparation, avoid aluminum pots and pans—excess aluminum has been found by some researchers in the brains of Alzheimer's patients. Limiting or eliminating your exposure to Teflon-coated pans is also a good idea, as the chemical used to make the nonstick substance is currently being studied for potential health risks. There's a reason why cast-iron pans were so popular with our grandparents. Moving back to them is not only safer for your health, it can make for better cooking results.

Finally, a word on cleaning products and kitchenware: Choose household and laundry cleaning alternatives that are less toxic than standard products, which contain harmful chemicals. Examples of less toxic cleaners include kosher soap, Citra Solv, Borax, That Orange Stuff and Nature Clean. For your laundry, consider non-toxic household products such as the ones by Seventh Generation.

HORMONE BOOST TIPS FOR KITCHEN TOOLS AND PREP

Jackie is a long-time team member at Clear Medicine, and it's widely known that she can cook! In light of her culinary skills, which we have all had the pleasure of experiencing at Christmas parties and lunch events, I asked her to compile some tips to guide you toward a kitchen setup that will further your success. These are her wonderful suggestions, backed by some of my own advice and information. But I have to admit, I picked up a new thing . . . or three . . .

Tools for Your Kitchen

- Invest in a set of sharp chef knives. As surprising as it sounds, sharp knives are safer than dull ones, since they are less likely to slip during use. And trust me, ready access to these essential tools will serve up simple satisfaction with every chop and slice.
- Get an immersion blender. This handy gadget will make puréeing dips, cauliflower mash and soups a breeze—and it will save you

dishes too, since your blending action can happen in the same pots used for cooking.

- Choose the right food processor (it can do wonders!). Food processors are great time-savers when it comes to chopping garlic or veggies. I have, and recommend, the Braun Multiquick System Handblender—it's a food processor, hand mixer and immersion blender all in one.

- Add a bench scraper to your utensil drawer. While it sounds like a tool you would find in a carpenter's kit, it's considered by many foodies and cooks to be a kitchen essential. This flat rectangular piece of metal with a handle across the full width of one edge might be the kitchen tool you never knew you needed—at least until you discover how useful it is. Use your scraper to transfer chopped ingredients from a cutting board with one steady swipe, crush garlic before peeling without the risk of cutting yourself, easily divide baking ingredients into halves, or slice cookie dough or veggies before cooking. You can also use it for lifting scraps into your green garbage bowl (where I suggest you hold scraps until disposal, thus saving time by avoiding frequent trips to the garbage).

- Savor the benefits of a slow cooker. Beyond the recipes I have shared with you in this book, there are a ton of healthy one-pot variations that make a busy family's dinner easily table-ready with little preparation time required. Ingredients can be prepped in the pot of the slow cooker and stored overnight in the fridge. In the morning, simply place the pot in the unit's base and turn it on. Most slow cookers take approximately eight hours to cook (when set on Low), which means a dish set out in the morning will be ready just in time for dinner. Working late? Some cookers have automatic timers that shut them off at the right time.

- Become reacquainted with a retro kitchen staple—the Mason jar. These traditional glass bottles are perfect for storing soups and sauces and for making the on-the-go salad recipes included in Chapter 14.

- Stock up on parchment paper. This, along with tinfoil, is an essential for any kitchen. Both come in handy for cooking fish fillets, veggies and meats. And both offer the bonus of making for easy cleanup.
- Consider making your home a microwave-free space. I rid myself of that nasty appliance years ago and replaced it with a high-quality toaster oven. Heating your food in the microwave can strip away its original nutrients. According to Dr. Joseph Mercola, an osteopathic doctor and an owner of one of the largest health websites in the world, originally healthy foods become "dead" from the dielectric heating in microwaves. The water molecules rotate rapidly in the microwave and in the food at high frequencies, which creates friction and heats up your food. This causes the molecular structure in your food to change and, as a result, diminishes the nutrient content in the food. A toaster oven is your best option for reheating leftovers or cooking meals for one, and it's the ideal way to prep my quiche muffin cups (page 270). Warm a serving from your frozen batch while getting ready in the morning, then grab it and go.
- Rely on stainless steel and glass bowls. These are fundamental in any kitchen. I have them in many sizes (mini ones for holding spices and large ones for prep work). They last a lifetime! It's an added bonus if you can find a set with lids, as they allow for easy fridge storage of dishes like salads or for marinating meats.
- Search for a spiralizer. Want to cut your carb intake or free yourself from the belly bloat of heavy pasta dishes? A spiralizer is your secret weapon for making virtually carb-free zucchini pasta and offers creative ways to increase your veggie intake (think cucumber, carrots and beets) in salads.
- Pick up a meat thermometer. A good meat thermometer ensures that roast chicken, beef and other meats are cooked through.

Staple Stock Items and Other Helpful Kitchen Tips

- Replace iodized table salt with Celtic sea salt. This natural option provides trace minerals that are beneficial for your thyroid, adrenal glands, body hydration, energy and overall wellness. It is available for purchase on my website if you can't find it at your local health food store.

- Stock your kitchen with a high-quality organic extra-virgin olive oil (contained in a dark bottle) and an organic coconut oil. These are also available in spray form at most health food stores—the perfect means for lightly glazing pans with just the right amount of oil.

- Buy low-sodium bouillon cubes, stocks and canned tomatoes.

- Substitute Greek yogurt for sour cream. It is lower in fat and higher in protein.

- You can enhance the flavor and depth of your meals without adding extra salt, using the acidity of vinegar (sherry, apple cider, balsamic) or lemon. An added benefit: Vinegars also reduce the glycemic impact of your meals.

- Prevent your cutting board from sliding by placing a damp paper towel underneath to hold it in place.

- Consider devoting one cupboard or drawer solely to the storage of your dry spices. Small glass jars are a perfect way to go—they're easy to label and arrange, and readily available at your local dollar store. Once you have your storage options in place, many spices can then be purchased in bulk.

- Firmly roll your lemons and limes against the counter surface to optimize the amount of juice you can extract from each fruit.

- When slicing avocados, use a sharp knife to split them in half and remove the pit. Then, keeping the skin intact, cut it into slices. This creates perfect sections, which can then be easily removed from the peel with a spoon, for use in salads and other dishes, or placed on a cookie sheet for freezing. Once the slices are frozen solid, transfer them to a sealed container or freezer bag.

- Always buy fresh fruits just before or at their peak and be sure to freeze them before they become too ripe. Take advantage of local farmers and picking seasons by stocking up on what's in season and freezing some for use in the winter months.

- Maintain the crispness of fresh herbs by washing, rolling in dampened paper towels and placing in resealable bags before storing in your fridge. Some fresh herbs can be washed and stored in your freezer to extend their shelf life for up to one month. Once frozen, they can be easily defrosted and chopped before they hit the pan.

- Here's a fresh idea for those with a green thumb: Prep a large planter and fill it with several herbs such as basil, mint, oregano and dill. I love harvesting the herbs at mealtimes; it makes me feel like I'm at home on my mom's farm in Nova Scotia.

- Always let your meats rest for at least five minutes after removing them from heat (roasts should rest for 10 to 20 minutes). This allows juices settled in the center of the meat to redistribute. Here's a specific chef's trick: Allow one minute of rest per 3.5 ounces of meat.

- When you make soup or sauces, drop an ice cube in your creation before finalizing your dish. The ice cube will attract fat and allow for its easy removal.

- Always read recipes from start to finish before starting to cook. This simple tip will help you visualize what's needed and in what order, and will ultimately help you improve your prep time. For example, you may realize that it's possible to cut all the veggies at once, regardless of when they are to be used, before moving on to use your cutting board for the meat in the recipe.

- Watch cooking shows! Everybody possesses the ability to cook, but observing new methods is part of what turns a cook into a chef (another part of that equation is lots and lots of practice!). Online or TV resources provide endless opportunities for learning on so many levels—from big-picture principles like the optimal temperature for cooking roast beef to the intricacies of which spices complement certain cuts of meat or stews.

- If you fail to plan, you plan to fail. Maximize your time management and success on the Hormone Boost by making an effort to plan your weekly meals. I shop and prep meals on Saturdays or Sundays, as often as possible. It keeps me on track and ensures that I have a full fridge for the week, when work or life becomes busy.
- Be present and enjoy your time in the kitchen. Make your food with the best of intentions. Holding this mindset will only enhance the health benefits of each and every meal. I love cooking on the weekends and when I have time—but I also understand that cooking often feels like work when you have so much on your plate already.
- Avoid mindless eating and overeating. Do this by making an effort to sit down at your table, free from the distractions of your phone, computer, tablet and TV.

Step Two: The Bathroom Boost

Most of us imagine our bathroom as an oasis—a place where we can soak in the tub or take a long, hot shower, washing away the stress of the day, and maybe pamper ourselves with a new skin-care or beauty product. But what happens when we take a closer look at those products? Think of all the stuff we slather on our skin or our hair, and then imagine how daily absorption of the chemicals in those products can add up over a lifetime. This long-term exposure is a definite hormonal and health concern. Some of the ingredients in beauty products aren't that pretty. In fact, according to the Environmental Working Group's cosmetic database (ewg.org), one in eight of the 82,000 ingredients used in personal care products are industrial chemicals, including carcinogens, pesticides, reproductive toxins and hormone disruptors. Imagine what that does to your skin, and to the environment.

Your cleansing products should be free of sodium lauryl sulphate (a harsh detergent present in shampoos and cleansers), and the products you use on your body and face should be free of all parabens (methylparabens, propylparabens, etc.), formaldehyde, imidazolidinyl urea, methylisothiazolinone, propylene glycol, paraffin, isopropyl alcohol and sodium lauryl sulphate. Most perfumed products contain many of these harmful chemicals, but the ingredients are not always identified on the label. To stay on the safe side, look for products that contain natural oils and fragrances.

Check out the list provided by Environmental Defence (environmentaldefence.ca) to help you avoid harmful chemicals in your cosmetics and skin-care products. Some ingredients (including phthalates, acrylamide, formaldehyde and ethylene oxide) are also listed by the U.S. Environmental Protection Agency and the state of California as a carcinogen risk.

Skin-Care Tips

- Pay close attention to the ingredients in every step of your skin-care routine. Avoid fragranced products, as they can be a problem for many people's skin. Even some essential oils like lavender or mint can be irritating, so gentle is the way to go when trying to repair your skin's barrier.
- Protect your skin from one of the most common causes of impaired barrier function: the sun. Use sunscreens that contain zinc and titanium (rather than chemicals) as active ingredients for sun protection, and apply often. My favorite sunscreen—a powder easy to apply to the face and body—is made by Colorescience.
- Use exfoliating products only two or three times per week, and choose ones that are free of harsh or rough particles, to avoid scratching the skin. Exfoliate only with those that containing acids (AHA, BHA or fruit acids like those in Green Apple Peel from Juice Beauty). They lift dead skin cells

instead of scraping them off. If you use retinol-based creams, apply them only at night.

- Many skin-care products actually damage the skin barrier (we'll chat more about the skin barrier in the next chapter) and clog detoxification pores, leading to a host of allergic conditions and other problems. Our skin eliminates waste to protect itself from toxins. It also accumulates toxins from products, which build up over time. Look for products that use natural active ingredients that are more "bio-identical." Here are a few effective options:

  > *Emollients:* Reinforce lipid barrier, lock in moisture, soften the skin and provide elasticity. Examples include jojoba oil, sweet almond oil, coconut oil and shea butter.

  > *Botanicals:* Provide skin-soothing properties and speed up the healing process. Try allantoin, aloe and colloidal oatmeal.

  > *Antioxidants:* Protect against environmental aggressors. Vitamins E and C are ideal for this.

  > *Minerals:* Essential for healthy skin function, they act as natural anti-inflammatory agents and provide relief against itching and redness (e.g., zinc oxide).

These ingredients provide healing and relief without the risk of the side effects associated with corticosteroids, which thin the skin, and without harmful chemical ingredients, such as parabens, that are linked to hormone disruption.

A few of my favorite brands and sources for natural skin-care products are:

- **Korres:** This company makes amazing body butters, lip balms and body lotions.
- **Naturopathica:** I love their Environmental Defense Mask. It's a natural fruit-acid mixture with a deep red color. It just looks and feels as if it is good for you.

- **Juice Beauty:** The Green Apple Peel is a fabulous exfoliant, and their new stem-cell moisturizer is fantastic.
- **Burt's Bees:** A wonderful array of products for the whole family.
- **Pure + Simple:** These stores carry a variety of natural skin-care brands.
- **SkinCeuticals:** I love their hyaluronic acid serum and vitamin C serum.
- **John Masters:** I adore the green tea and vitamin C facial serums, Blood Orange & Vanilla Body Milk and all of their shampoos and conditioners.
- As a natural alternative to perfume, use body oils that are scented with natural essential oils. Look for Young Living Essential Oils or doTERRA oils.

Step Three: The Bedroom Boost

The final step in your Hormone Boost home preparation comes—you guessed it—in the bedroom. No surprise, really, given what we learned in Part One about the importance of sleep. Not only does poor sleep pack on pounds, good sleep actually helps you to lose weight by influencing the hormones that control your appetite and increase your metabolism. A 2004 study at the University of Chicago was the first to show sleep as a major regulator of appetite-controlling hormones. It also linked the extent of hormonal variations with the degree of hunger change. More specifically, researchers found that, among subjects who were sleep deprived, *appetite-enhancing ghrelin* increased by 28 percent, while *appetite-curbing leptin* decreased by 18 percent. Appetite is not the only factor that increases with lack of sleep—the desire for high-calorie, high-sugar foods also jumps.

In 2004, researchers at the Stanford University School of Medicine found that subjects who got only five hours of sleep per night had less leptin and more ghrelin *and* experienced an increase in their

BMI, *regardless of diet and exercise.* Let's face it—no one feels good after endless nights of tossing, turning or staring at the ceiling.

Ask yourself the following questions:

- Do I fall asleep as soon as my head hits the pillow?
- Do I rely on an alarm to wake me up?
- Do I feel tired during the day?
- Do I tend to sleep more on the weekends?

If you answered yes to all of the above, you are probably sleep deprived. Sleep deprivation perpetuates a vicious cycle of excessive stress hormones, reduced sleep-inducing melatonin and low growth hormone. Your hormonal state also influences your ability to sleep. For instance, hormonal imbalances associated with PMS or the low serotonin common with depression can lead to many frustrating nights of tossing and turning or repeatedly waking in the wee morning hours.

The look, feel, temperature, lighting and sound in your bedroom can either help or hinder your sleep. So before you even hit the pillow, you have to make sure your space is set up to promote healthy sleep. Here are a few suggestions to help you get started:

- **Make your room as dark as possible**. When you hit the hay, you should not be able to see your hand in front of your face. If you must use an alarm clock, turn it away from you. I use blackout curtains and recommend that my patients do the same. Your children should also sleep in the dark. If they're afraid of the dark, try turning off the night-light after they've drifted off to sleep. Why make your room a den of darkness? Because when light hits your skin, it disrupts the circadian rhythm of the pineal gland and, as a result, hinders the production of melatonin. Studies have shown that even a small amount of light can cause a decrease in melatonin levels—and that affects sleep, interferes with weight loss and may raise your cancer risk.

- **Use low lighting in your bedroom.** Once you settle into bed, avoid using overhead lights and lamps with high-wattage bulbs. My husband and I have replaced our overhead light fixture with a ceiling fan, and we each use our own clip-on or handheld book lights for reading. These are great for lighting only the page and not shining in your eyes or illuminating the entire room, which can potentially interfere with your sleep or your partner's.

- **Be aware of electromagnetic fields (EMFs).** These can disrupt the pineal gland and the production of melatonin and serotonin. They may have additional negative effects, including an increased risk of cancer. EMFs are emitted from digital alarm clocks and other electrical devices. If you must use these items, try to keep them as far away from the bed as possible—at least three feet.

- **Turn off the TV; turn on your love life.** Television is another source of hormone-disrupting EMFs. Studies show that you will enjoy better sleep and more of it without a TV in the bedroom. Besides, you're also likely to have more sex when you ban the TV from your sleep space. And the better your hormonal health, the more often you will have enjoyable sex. (Not having sex actually causes hormonal imbalance. The "use it or lose it" rule applies here!) If you must watch TV simply to turn your mind off at the end of the day, use the timer function to make sure the set goes off if you fall asleep. That way you'll never be wakened by the noise and light from the TV. Also, keep the television at least six feet from the bed.

- **Use your bed only for sleeping, light reading (from a book, not a Kindle!) and sex.** If you have kids, you know how easily your bedroom can become Grand Central Station for the entire family. But you should definitely avoid engaging in any other activities in bed, because you may start to associate the bedroom with sleep-robbing chores and tasks rather than relaxing sleep and intimacy with your partner. Above all, never work in bed.

- **Create bedroom "zen."** In my last two homes, I painted the bedroom calming dark, earthy tones. Shades like these help make the bedroom a relaxing place. Over the years, I've also realized that clutter is a state of mind. Keeping your bedroom neat and clutter-free can be challenging, especially if you live in a small space. Just remember, the primary purpose of the bedroom is sleep and sex. You'll be amazed how much better both will be if you try to keep your bedside tables and dresser tops clear of clutter.

- **Choose comfortable, soothing bedding.** Several companies now offer organic cotton bedding lines that are free of harmful dyes and toxins. These can be a great investment if you have sensitive skin or simply care about the impact of heavy pesticide use on the environment. Personally, I find all-white bedding very soothing and welcoming after a long day of sensory overload. Whatever your taste dictates, select bedding that pleases your eye and feels good on your skin. You should also make sure your bedding keeps you warm but doesn't overheat you. In the winter you may wish to use a duvet, while a thin blanket with a sheet might suffice for summer. Small changes like these will help create a calming, comfortable environment conducive to restful sleep.

- **Keep your bedroom cool but not cold.** No matter how chilly the weather gets outside, your bedroom temperature should be no warmer than 70°F (21°C) for sleeping. Remember, our body needs to cool slightly at night to ensure proper release of our sleep-inducing hormone, melatonin. At the same time, make sure your air conditioner is not blasting all night long in the summertime. Research shows that air conditioning can cause weight gain.

- **Consider purchasing a white-noise device**. If you live in an apartment building or noisy neighborhood, you're probably familiar with the aggravation of being awakened by sounds. You may even wake when your partner walks around at night or snores. If you find you are easily awakened by sounds, the hum of a white-noise machine or a household fan may help. You can also try wearing earplugs.

- **Avoid using a loud alarm clock**. Waking up suddenly to the blaring wail of an alarm clock can be a shock to your body; you'll find you feel groggier when you are roused in the middle of a sleep cycle. Getting enough sleep on a regular basis should make your alarm clock unnecessary. In fact, sleeping through an alarm or relying on an alarm daily may indicate that you are sleep deprived. If you do use an alarm, you should awaken just before it goes off. If you must use one, I recommend the Bose clock radio. It starts off at a moderate volume and slowly gets louder, so you aren't jarred out of your sleep. You can also look into getting a sunrise alarm clock, which wakes you with gradually increasing light that simulates a sunrise. This method of waking has the added bonus of improving your mood and increasing your energy throughout the day.

- **If you go to the bathroom during the night, keep the lights off**. Even brief exposure to light can shut down the melatonin production that's so crucial for good sleep. If you absolutely must use a light in the bathroom, try a flashlight or night-light instead of the bright overhead light. Another option is to use a dimmer switch or a night-light fitted with a red bulb, since red light exposure at night appears to have less of a negative impact.

- **Invest in a comfortable mattress**. Your mattress should be comfortable for you and your partner—not too hard or too soft. When my mom starting having hip and shoulder pain, we looked at a number of factors and finally came to the conclusion that her mattress was too hard. As soon as she changed it to a pillow-top mattress, the problem was solved. The right degree of firmness or softness is a personal thing, and your preference may change with age (just like my mom's).

  A note about the chemicals in mattresses: In an effort to reduce the number of deaths or injuries caused by mattress fires ignited by cigarettes, a standard was enacted in 1973 calling for preventive measures. This resulted in flame-retardant chemicals being added to mattresses, such as boric acid and antimony, decabromodiphenyl oxide, zinc borate, melamine, PBDEs, PVC and formaldehyde. Unfortunately, these same flame-retardant chemicals are linked to cancer, SIDS, prenatal mortality, reduced fertility, neurological disorders and other negative effects. You may wish to look for a chemical-free wool mattress.

  Products from IKEA and Essentia are chemical free, while Sealy and Serta are in the process of making changes to their mattresses, though they don't yet completely meet safety standards. If you have already invested in a quality mattress but are unsure of its chemical content, an activated carbon blanket can reduce your exposure to toxic mattress fumes (visit www.nontoxic.com).
- **No pets or kids**! Sleeping with your pet(s) or children may disrupt your precious sleep. Have them sleep in their own bed instead.

Once you've turned your bedroom into a healthy, sleep-inducing oasis, the next critical step is to start sleeping correctly. You may not have known that *there is actually a proper way and time to sleep.*

It's true! When, how and how much we sleep is important. Failing to follow these recommendations can impede the fat-burning and hormone-balancing benefits you should gain from sleep each and every night. These simple rules help to boost testosterone, thyroid, growth hormone, melatonin, serotonin, dopamine and DHEA!

- **Sleep in complete darkness.** As I explained earlier in this section, even a small amount of light can hamper your sleep.
- **Sleep nude (or at least with loose-fitting nightclothes—but nude is better).** Do not sleep in tight undergarments (bras, girdles, briefs, etc.). Tight clothing will increase your body temperature and interfere with melatonin release while you sleep.
- **Establish regular sleeping hours.** Try to get up each morning and go to bed every night at roughly the same time. Over-sleeping can be as detrimental as sleep deprivation. How you feel each day is an important indication of how much sleep is right for you.
- **Get to bed by 11 p.m.** Since the invention of electricity (not to mention television, computers and smartphones), we have begun staying up later and later. This change has resulted in a largely sleep-deprived society. Our stress glands—the adrenals—recharge or recover most between 11 p.m. and 1 a.m. Going to bed before 11 p.m. (in fact, 10 p.m. is even better) is optimal for rebuilding your adrenal reserves. I know this can be difficult to change, so I recommend to my patients that they start going to bed 15 minutes earlier each week until they reach their new target time.
- **Sleep 7.5 to 9 hours a night.** The American Cancer Society has found higher incidences of cancer in individuals who consistently sleep less than six hours or more than nine hours nightly. Consistently needing more than nine hours of sleep every night warrants a visit to your doctor for further

investigation, as this may indicate an underlying medical condition such as hypothyroidism, depression or a deficiency of iron, folic acid or vitamin B_{12}. Some of us simply require more or less sleep than others. If you awake without an alarm and feel rested, you're likely getting the right amount of sleep for you.

- **See the light first thing in the morning.** Daylight and morning sounds are key signals that help awaken your brain. Turning on the lights or opening the blinds is the proper way to reset your body clock and ensure that your melatonin level drops back to "awake" mode until the evening. Exposure to morning light has also been proven to be one of the simplest ways to increase your energy for the entire day. It's been shown to boost testosterone in men and fertility in women by stimulating luteinizing hormone release from the pituitary gland. Enhance this action further by exposing yourself to sunlight and by getting outside during the day. I can't say enough about the benefits of getting outside, even for 10 to 20 minutes, in the morning light.
- **Keep household lighting dim from dinnertime until you go to sleep.** Believe it or not, this simple step not only prepares your body and hormones for sleep, but it also helps your digestion.
- **Use natural sleep aids when needed.** If you find you need additional remedies to help improve your sleep, try one or more of these:
  > **Clear Balance – Stress Modifying Formula.** This contains Relora, my favourite choice for chronic stress and sleep disruption. And boy, does it work! A mixture of tree extracts from *Magnolia officinalis* and *Phellodendron amurense*, Relora is medically proven to reduce stress and anxiety. It's often the best option for patients who tend to wake up throughout the night, for highly stressed individuals and for menopausal women with hot flashes that cause sleep

disruption. Relora can significantly reduce cortisol and raise the anti-aging, anti-stress hormone DHEA within only two weeks of use. Take two capsules before bed and one in the morning to ease the effects of stress and improve your rest. Alternatively, you can take all three at night. This product works very well when combined with melatonin.

> **Magnesium glycinate.** This simple mineral works so well that I once had a patient question whether I had given him a drug for his sleep! Magnesium calms your nervous system, induces relaxation, reduces blood pressure, decreases cravings, aids PMS tension, increases energy during the day, and treats and prevents constipation and muscle cramps. As an added bonus, it also reduces sugar cravings and aids insulin sensitivity. It's truly one of nature's "wonder drugs." Take 200 to 800 mg at night. Begin at 200 mg and keep increasing the dosage until you reach bowel tolerance (i.e., the point at which you develop loose stools). Topical magnesium chloride gel is also an excellent way to increase your magnesium stores, improve sleep and calm your nervous system. Use one application on each limb at bedtime. A second application after your shower in the morning can also be used.

> **Ashwagandha.** Ayurvedic practitioners use this dietary supplement to enhance mental and physical performance, improve learning ability and decrease stress and fatigue. Ashwagandha is a general tonic that can be used in stressful situations, especially for insomnia, restlessness or when you are feeling overworked. Studies have indicated that ashwagandha offers anti-inflammatory, anti-cancer, anti-stress, antioxidant and immune-modulating and rejuvenating properties. The typical dosage is 500 to 1,000 mg twice daily. Capsules should be standardized to 1.5 percent withanolides per dose. My favorite brand is AOR.

> **GABA.** Gamma-aminobutyric acid (GABA) is an inhibitory neurotransmitter, a brain chemical that has a calming effect. It's well suited for individuals who experience anxiety, muscle tension or pain. Take 500 to 1,000 mg before bed. Alternatively, take GABA 10 to 20 minutes before your evening meal. The standard dose of 500 mg twice daily can be increased to a maximum of three times daily if needed, but this dosage should not be exceeded. You can also consider Clear Calm – GABA Enhancing Formula or GABA 500 mg capsules from Douglas Labs.

> **Clear Mood (contains 5-HTP).** A derivative of tryptophan that also contributes to the creation of serotonin, 5-HTP has been found to be more effective than tryptophan in treating sleep loss related to depression, anxiety and fibromyalgia. It also appears to increase REM sleep and decrease the amount of time required to fall asleep and the number of nighttime awakenings. And remember, the higher your serotonin, the less your risk of carb cravings. Take 50 to 400 mg a day, divided into doses throughout the day and before bed. Clear Mood – Serotonin Support Formula works very well because it also contains the vitamin cofactors needed for production of serotonin, along with 75 mg of 5-HTP per capsule.

> **Melatonin.** This hormone decreases as we age, as well as during times of stress and depression. Take 0.5 to 3 mg at bedtime. You should purchase melatonin in sublingual or lozenge form, rather than pills or capsules, for best absorption. Supplements tend to be effective for insomnia only when melatonin levels are low, so if you find it doesn't work for you, this could be the reason. Use Clear ZZZ's – Melatonin lozenges. They're really potent and work fast! I feel groggy about 20 minutes after taking one.

Once these simple steps for your home have been completed, you are ready to take the simple steps for your body—specifically your digestion, liver, skin and libido.

A HORMONE BOOST REAL-LIFE SUCCESS STORY

THE CLIENTS: The dynamic duo—Sharon and Ross

BODY COMPOSITION RESULTS (FROM SCALE AND BODY FAT/ MUSCLE MASS VIA BIO-IMPEDANCE TESTING)

SHARON: Age 56

MEASUREMENT	BEFORE	AFTER	TOTAL LOSS/GAIN
Weight (lb.)	101	105	(+) 4
Lean Body Mass (lb.)	74.4	80.4	(+) 6
Fat Mass (lb.)	26.6	24.6	(-) 2
Basal Metabolic Rate (calories/day)	1051 calories	1136 calories	(+) 85

ROSS: Age 57

MEASUREMENT	BEFORE	AFTER	TOTAL LOSS/GAIN
Weight (lb.)	188	186	(-) 2
Lean Body Mass (lb.)	145.1	145.5	(+) 0.4
Fat Mass (lb.)	42.9	40.5	(-) 2.4
Basal Metabolic Rate (calories/day)	2053 calories	2079 calories	(+) 26

After attending a speaking engagement in Calgary, Sharon and Ross came to my clinic and immediately became two of my favorite patients. They arrived in good health, with limited ailments and the goal of optimizing their overall wellness.

Sharon's initial concerns were fatigue and a desire to address her low bone density, while my initial case intake with Ross revealed arthritis in his ankles as his sole complaint.

These dynamos exhibited a healthy bit of competition as they jointly embarked on their detox, mastering the rules of hormonally balanced nutrition and sticking to their daily supplement prescriptions. And they both enjoyed favorable outcomes as a result. Ross experienced complete removal of the arthritic pain in his ankles and Sharon was feeling stronger and more energized. Although her biannual bone-density test results are still pending, she continues to embrace the essential lifestyle habits for her bone health. I think we can safely conclude that the six-pound gain in her lean body mass noted in the interim proves it!

CHAPTER 9

FOUR-STEP BODY PREP

Believe in yourself! Have faith in your abilities!
Without a humble but reasonable confidence in your
own powers you cannot be successful or happy.

NORMAN VINCENT PEALE

Now that you've cruised through the simple steps for your home, it's time to focus on your body. Are you ready to optimize the fat-loss six by optimizing your digestion, activating liver function, using sex for a hormone boost and protecting your skin barrier? (Yes, I just said "using sex for a hormone boost!") These four prep steps are your essential building blocks.

Step One: Give Your Digestion a Boost

Does it surprise you to hear that your digestive system is the largest hormone-producing tissue in your body? The hormones produced within the gut have an effect on digestion as well as the entire body—including the brain, immune system, pancreas and liver. For instance, although serotonin is well known as a brain neuro-transmitter, it is estimated that 90 percent of the body's serotonin is actually made in the digestive tract. In fact, altered levels of this peripheral serotonin have been linked to irritable bowel syndrome, cardiovascular disease and osteoporosis.

It makes sense that what you see on your belly essentially begins with what's in your mouth, but it can also be impacted by what's *in* your belly. The health of your digestive system and beneficial gut flora (otherwise known as probiotics) influences the number of calories that are absorbed from your food and stored in your body. The carbohydrates you eat are broken down into sugar through the process of digestion, which begins in the mouth and ends in your small intestine. From there, what's going on in your gut has a huge impact on your metabolic function and your ability to break down toxins, synthesize nutrients, process indigestible food, regulate the immune system and produce the hormones needed to appropriately direct the storage of fat.

Research from the Mayo Clinic (April 2008) has linked favorable intestinal bacteria with the ability to get slim and stay that way. The metabolic activities of gut flora facilitate extraction of calories from the foods eaten and help to store those calories in fat tissue for later use. Furthermore, researchers found that the bacterial gut flora of obese mice and humans includes more types of calorie-storing bacteria than that of their lean counterparts. These findings suggest that gut flora may play a key role in regulating weight. The human body, which consists of about 100 trillion cells, carries about ten times that many microorganisms in the intestines and GI tract. And anything that affects nutritional absorption impacts caloric expenditure.

Ready for another surprise? A whopping 60 to 70 percent of our immune system is clustered around our digestive tract. That's why improving digestive health and avoiding digestion-compromising factors—including food allergies, a deficiency of beneficial gut flora (intestinal bacteria) or an overgrowth of harmful bacteria, deficiency of enzymes or acids, yeast overgrowth, parasites and stress—are important not only to the digestive process itself but to the entire immune system. Painful conditions such as gas, bloating, heartburn, reflux, constipation, diarrhea, irritable bowel syndrome,

Crohn's disease and ulcerative colitis are *all* related to inflammation in the digestive system and hormonal imbalance.

Moreover, keeping your bowels moving properly will help to ensure that waste does not build up in your body, create toxicity or

---

The Transit-Time Test

Normal transit time for food passing through your intestines is about 18 to 24 hours. If it takes longer than 24 hours, there is something off with your digestive system. Try this easy at-home test to see how your system is performing:

- Purchase a product called activated charcoal, an inert substance that will turn your stool black or dark gray. You can purchase this product at health food stores.
- Swallow four capsules with a meal and write down the day and time.
- Observe your stool until you see black or dark gray stool appear. When this happens, write down the day and time. Compare this to the time at which you originally swallowed the capsules.
- If it took longer than 24 hours for the black or dark gray stool to appear, you have some work to do on your digestive tract. If it took

less than 18 hours, that may also signal a problem: there is something irritating the digestive tract that could be causing increased peristalsis (wave-like contractions in the digestive system to promote movement), such as bacterial imbalance, inflammation or food allergies.

Comprehensive Stool Testing

The best way to determine if you have problems in your digestive tract is to complete a comprehensive stool analysis. I recommend testing through the Doctor's Data laboratory (doctorsdata.com); I have been using them for years. Their comprehensive stool analysis tests for harmful bacteria overgrowth, parasites, infections, inflammation, probiotic balance, blood, mucus and even how well you digest your protein, carbs and fats. It also tells you which natural and pharmaceutical agents will be suitable to counteract detected imbalances.

Two Digestive Tests

hamper your overall health. This simple activity also helps to prevent a buildup of estrogen by-products, since estrogen is metabolized in the liver and excreted into the digestive system in the bile. Bacteria in the large bowel further aid the breakdown of estrogen. Liver function, bile secretion, bacterial balance and sufficient bowel movements are essential to ridding the body of toxins, especially excess estrogen, which can increase cancer risks.

If you are having digestive problems, there is a good chance that it is affecting your mood, immunity and so much more (including thyroid hormone function). Bloating after meals, gas, cramping, loose stools, constipation, burping, heartburn and inconsistent stool formation can all be signs of a digestive problem. If this is your experience, I recommend you follow my tips for a digestive boost.

Tips for a Digestive Boost
Use these basic suggestions to give your digestion a boost:

- **Consistently take a probiotic** (e.g., Clear Flora) upon rising or before bed.
- **Try increasing your fiber**—but choose the right type to suit your digestive needs. I recommend Herbulk (made by Metagenics), or a product with similar ingredients, for those of you prone to loose stools. Clear Fiber, a hypoallergenic fiber supplement, is a great choice to combat constipation and improve bowel regularity—it really should be considered an essential staple in this plan. Add your chosen fiber supplement to smoothies or mix it in water before meals or bedtime.
- **Get and keep things moving**. Ideal bowel function is one to three times per day. I once said on the *Marilyn Denis Show,* "It's all about poopin' and sleepin'." Isn't that the truth? We really can't optimize our hormones unless waste is cleared out and we are free of belly bloat. I commonly prescribe

magnesium at bedtime to treat (and prevent) constipation—
it's a favorite option because it helps sleep too. Start with one
capsule at bedtime and increase nightly until you reach the
"sweet spot" (you'll know when you've gone past it!). A powdered vitamin C supplement called Effer-C (from Douglas
Labs) is the best remedy I've found for stubborn chronic
constipation, and it can be used in combination with magnesium. This product's specific blend of minerals is what
makes it work so well. Begin with half a teaspoon in a small
amount of water at bedtime. Do not exceed more than one
teaspoon at a time. And a heads-up: It doesn't taste good,
so I recommend you limit your suffering by mixing it with
just a small amount of water and shooting it down. You can
find both these products online in my Supercharge Your
Digestion Kit.

- **Consider following the first three weeks of my Supercharged
Hormone Diet plan.** My book *The Supercharged Hormone
Diet* will help you identify your food sensitivities and reduce
inflammation in the gut. Then return to your Hormone
Boost for week 4 and beyond, free of your food sensitivities.

Step Two: Give Your Liver Some Love

Everything you breathe, eat or absorb through your skin ends up in
your bloodstream and eventually passes through your liver. It is
your primary detoxifier and fat-burning organ, so keeping it healthy
is critical to your Hormone Boost, because of its influence on your
metabolism, as well as its activation of and effect on the fat-loss six.

I often tell my patients that I think they would be a lot nicer to
their liver if it were on their face! Our liver operates like a waste
treatment plant (sounds sexy, doesn't it?). It takes everything we
put into our bodies—or that gains access via the skin or lungs—
and filters it. That process separates the nutrients needed for energy
and other bodily functions from waste products. It then helps to

dispose of what we do not need, including the by-products of metabolism, hormonal waste and toxins.

But there are so many other things your liver does for you:

- It converts fats, proteins and carbohydrates to energy and nutrients.
- It creates bile to break down fats and eliminate fat-soluble toxins and potentially harmful excess hormones, such as estrogen.
- It helps to regulate sex hormone balance and manufacture testosterone and estrogen.
- It activates thyroid hormone and supports growth hormone activation and function.
- It metabolizes drugs, alcohol and chemicals.
- It stores vitamins and minerals, such as iron (ferritin) and vitamin B_{12}, as well as sugars as fuel (glycogen) for future use.
- It helps maintain fluid and electrolyte balance.
- It creates serum proteins that act as hormone carriers.
- It creates immune substances such as gamma globulin.
- It filters blood, regulates blood clotting and stores extra blood for quick release.
- It plays a vital role in the body's use of hormones, both those that are produced naturally in our bodies and those that are introduced via hormone therapies.

Supporting the detoxification processes in the liver requires many nutrients and sufficient protein intake, which provides the amino acids needed at various stages of detoxification. If these nutrients are in short supply, the liver cannot process as quickly or as thoroughly as needed. When this happens, the toxins or waste buildup can escape back into the body, leading to serious health concerns and metabolic disruption.

For example, the Phase I pathway is the main metabolic pathway for the estrogen hormones. In premenopausal women, the ovaries produce estrogen, primarily estradiol, most of which the body converts to estrone (the "harmful" estrogen) and eventually estriol (the "good" estrogen). The liver then metabolizes the remaining estradiol and the converted estrone, breaking it down further and excreting the excess from the body.

Phase I processing can be affected by many factors, including the effects of alcohol or drugs, a lack of nutrients, or interference from other substances. Grapefruit juice, for instance, can slow down the enzymes in Phase I, potentially altering hormone balance. And many prescription drugs are metabolized in Phase I, which can also interfere with the liver's ability to handle the estrogen hormones.

On the other hand, indole-3-carbinol (I3C), a phytonutrient derived from cruciferous vegetables (e.g., broccoli, cauliflower, cabbage and Brussels sprouts), stimulates the enzymes that promote the metabolism of estrogens into milder forms, potentially reducing the risk of estrogen-dependent cancers. I3C is an essential ingredient in a product I suggest taking during your Hormone Boost: Clear Detox – Hormonal Health.

During Phase II, a process known as conjugation begins, in which nutrients such as amino acids are combined with hormones and other substances to convert them to water-soluble compounds that can be excreted efficiently in the urine or stool. Of the various processes that may occur in Phase II, the following are most relevant to hormone metabolism:

- **Methylation** is the process in which small parts of molecules, called methyl groups, are passed from one molecule to another. Once estrogens are methylated, they can be easily excreted. In order for the liver to have an adequate supply of methyl groups, an adequate intake of vitamins B_6, B_{12} and folic acid is necessary. I have included all of these nutrients for you in Clear Detox – Hormonal Health.

- **Sulfation** is the process in which sulfur groups are added to estrogen or other molecules to prepare them for easy excretion. Adequate amounts of foods containing sulfur should be in the diet, including egg yolks, garlic, onions and Brussels sprouts. Animal protein is another important source of sulfur.

- **Glucuronidation** is another process by which estrogens can be conjugated. This type of conjugation may be affected by the condition of the intestines. If the intestines have an abundance of abnormal bacteria, an enzyme produced by these bacteria may cut off the conjugated part from the estrogen. The estrogen that would have been excreted is then reabsorbed back into the body, which allows even estrogens produced by the body to build up to excessive levels. The calcium-D-glucarate naturally found in some fruits and vegetables and in supplement form, however, can render the enzyme inactive and prevent this buildup. That's why it's a main ingredient in Clear Detox – Hormonal Health.

- **Glutathione conjugation** is the process in which glutathione, another sulfur-containing molecule, is added to estrogen for easy excretion. Foods such as whey protein, avocado, walnuts and asparagus are rich in glutathione. Vitamin C also stimulates the body to produce more of it. Glutathione depletion can be caused by a lack of the essential nutrients and amino acids (found in fresh fruits, vegetables, fish and meats) needed to synthesize it.

Liver function and hormone balance are intimately connected, because liver function has a critical effect on hormones and, at the same time, is affected by hormones—the ones produced in the body as well as those used as therapy. So be kind to your liver!

Reduce its burden whenever possible; avoid overeating and heavy alcohol intake, and provide adequate supplies of nutrients to assist detoxification, with the complete Hormone Boost diet plan—which is rich in fiber and healthy fats and low in carbohydrates. Drink plenty of water to facilitate the elimination of toxic and excess substances. And, finally, since your liver is so dependent on many nutrients to complete its job of breaking down and removing any excess toxins, as well as activating other hormones, include Clear Detox – Hormonal Health or a similar product (you can view all of the ingredients online). Lovin' your liver like this is key to your Hormone Boost.

THREE WAYS TO BEAT STRESS AND GET A HORMONE BOOST: MEDITATION, MASSAGE AND LAUGHTER

Even when we know what and how much we are supposed to eat, emotional factors and stress greatly influence our food choices and consumption. Eating can be a very pleasurable, often social, experience, closely tied to feelings and emotions. Many of us use food for comfort or to cope with stressful, upsetting situations, especially when we have not developed more effective coping strategies. We also eat when we're bored, feel like celebrating, want to boost our spirits or are avoiding dealing with anxiety, fear, anger and resentment. In the very short term, food can make us feel good. But over the long haul, stress-related eating can leave us with feelings of guilt and regret, not to mention excess pounds. You can, however, use meditation, massage and laughter to reduce stress-related eating.

Meditation

Meditation has amazing effects on your hormones, lowering the stress hormones cortisol and adrenaline and raising the anti-aging, anti-stress hormones DHEA and serotonin. The only requirement is discipline and the ability to comfortably spend a few moments alone without distractions. Once you incorporate it into your daily routine, you'll find that the journey to enlightenment is accompanied by endless physical, emotional and spiritual benefits.

How to Meditate in Six Simple Steps

1. **Get comfortable.** Sit or lie in a comfortable, quiet place where you will not be interrupted or distracted. You may want to designate a space at home for this.

2. **Clear your mind.** Close your eyes, rest and *do nothing*.

3. **Concentrate on your breath.** Focus on the sound of your breathing, how it feels flowing in and out at the edges of your nostrils. I find it useful to imagine my breath washing in and out like waves on a beach. You can also pick a word or a phrase that is soothing or meaningful to you. One patient of mine, an extremely tense 85-year-old man with high blood pressure, picked the word *quiet*, which I thought was a great choice. Repeat the word or phrase to yourself each time you exhale.

4. **Practice body awareness.** Check for tension, especially in your jaw, scalp, forehead, shoulders, lower back and hips—all the way down to your toes—by consciously examining each body part. Relax the areas that feel tight, as you continue breathing.

5. **Stay in tune with your breathing or the repetition of your word or phrase.** You'll be amazed at how often thoughts start creeping back into your mind. Just acknowledge them and return your focus to your breathing. With practice, the amount of time you'll be able to sit without your mind wandering will lengthen, and you may even find that solutions you've been searching for will appear.

6. **Can't get your focus into the present?** Close your eyes and ask yourself, "What do I hear right now?" Attaching your attention to a sense will allow you to become "in the moment" and will put an end to your mind's dwelling on the past or worrying about the future. This simple exercise keeps you right here, right now. Try it.

Some forms of meditation may involve repetitive physical motions such as running or cycling. If you want to meditate while engaging in these activities, practice staying focused on your breathing and allowing your thoughts to flow freely. This form of meditation is very helpful for people who have a difficult time sitting still.

Massage

More than just an enjoyable indulgence, massage offers a host of health benefits that can help our weight-loss efforts. A study from the *International Journal of Neuroscience* (October 2005) found that massage increases endorphin release, which is excellent for treating pain, depression and anxiety. Massage also helps ease activity in the sympathetic nervous system (responsible for our fight-or-flight response) and increases our parasympathetic response (which induces us to rest and relax).

Moreover, we know that the cortisol and adrenaline we produce when we're under stress are destructive to our body tissues, immune system and adrenal glands when they are present in high amounts for long periods of time. One of the liver's functions is to break down stress and sex hormones. Massage, which assists the blood flow and lymphatic delivery of hormonal waste to the liver, expedites this process, thereby helping to relieve stress in the body.

Remember, anything that reduces our sympathetic nervous system's responses can help propel weight loss, ease water retention and boost appetite control. So massage has definite physiological benefits beyond simply feeling good while you are on the table.

Laughter

I once prescribed watching the movie *Planes, Trains and Automobiles* to a 65-year-old woman who was constantly worried about her health. I also told a diabetic man of 35, "Don't come back here unless you've done something *fun*." I kid you not. Genuine laughter can relieve stress and improve health. Professor Lee S. Berk of Loma

Linda University in California has found that *the mere anticipation of laughter* has significant positive hormonal effects. In a recent study, one group of subjects was told they were about to watch a funny movie, while the second group was told that they would be reading magazines for an hour. When tested, those who were told about the movie had 27 percent more beta-endorphins and 87 percent more growth hormone. In previous studies, Berk found that laughter reduced cortisol and adrenaline and enhanced the immune system for 12 to 24 hours. So, watch funny movies and make time for laughter in your life—or just think about doing it!

Step Three: Give Your Sex Life a Boost (and Get a Hormone Boost!)

Sexual function is a lot like lean muscle—if we don't use it, we lose it *and* the health and hormonal benefits that come with it. Guys, if your sex life is in the doldrums lately, you likely have less testosterone as well. The fix is pretty straightforward, though. Research shows that if we can get you back to enjoying more frequent sex, your testosterone can, ahem, rise again. A group of Italian researchers looked at men with erectile issues and measured their testosterone status before and after treatment (though not with testosterone replacement). Those whose treatment was successful had higher testosterone compared with those whose treatments failed to yield improvements. If you needed a strong argument for having sex tonight, now you have one.

Ladies, the same principles apply to you. Women who enjoy more lovin' in the bedroom have increased estrogen and testosterone. When present in the proper balance, these hormones add fire to sexual desire, give us more sex appeal, improve mood and memory and can even prevent abdominal fat gain. A little precoital cuddling, however, is also very important. Scientists at Simon Fraser University (February 2008) measured the level of testosterone in women before and after sex, cuddling and exercise. Their study results, published in the journal *Hormones and Behavior*, showed that although the women's testosterone was higher both before and after sexual intercourse, cuddling gave them the biggest testosterone boost of all.

I have seen thousands of men with andropause (caused by a drop in testosterone) and women with PMS, irregular periods, perimenopause or menopause (caused by a decrease or imbalance of estrogen or progesterone) in my office over the past 15 years, all in need of a sex hormone boost for optimal fertility, libido, memory, cognition, mood and sleep. And then there's the belly fat.

According to projections by the Government of Canada, one in six women will hit menopause within the next decade. Contrary to popular belief, menopause, which can begin as early as 40, is not just about estrogen decline. So many women come to my office intensely frustrated by the unwelcome changes in their body, especially an annoying thickening of the waistline. Other common symptoms of menopause include hot flashes, difficulty sleeping, headaches, heart palpitations, poor memory and concentration, urinary urgency or incontinence, vaginal dryness, changes in the appearance of their skin and hair and emotional changes that include depression, anxiety and irritability.

Testosterone enhances libido, bone density, muscle mass, strength, motivation, memory, fat burning and skin tone in both men and women. An increase in body fat and loss of muscle may happen, even with dieting and exercise, when testosterone is low. Testosterone levels tend to taper off with aging, obesity and stress, but today men are experiencing testosterone decline much earlier in life. This is an alarming finding, considering that low testosterone has been linked to depression, obesity, osteoporosis, heart disease—even death. Dr. Mitchell Harman, an endocrinologist at the University of Arizona College of Medicine, blames the proliferation of endocrine-suppressing estrogen-like compounds in pesticides and other farming chemicals for the downward trend in male testosterone levels. Phthalates, commonly found in cosmetics, soaps and most plastics, are another known cause of testosterone suppression.

For those of you who might be struggling in these life phases, I suggest that you bolster your Hormone Boost by implementing the following specific tips; they will help you restore sex hormone balance. Both guys and ladies can use all the recommendations provided elsewhere in this book for a testosterone boost to fuel fat burning and improve strength. But specifically for you, ladies, include a few of the suggestions below for symptoms of estrogen and progesterone imbalance.

Dietary Suggestions

- **Pay attention to food selections.** When selecting protein, carb, fat and fiber, go for options that are also high in phytoestrogens, such as fermented soy, legumes, pomegranate, fennel and flaxseeds. Phytoestrogens can help to improve low estrogen symptoms like hot flashes, night sweats, cravings and depression.
- **If you have breast tenderness or hot flashes**, completely avoid caffeine and alcohol for at least two weeks. After that, keep alcohol to a minimum—one to two drinks maximum, two to three days a week—and coffee to one cup in the morning. If the hot flashes or breast tenderness return or worsen, I recommend removing these foods from your diet again. Unlike my other books, *The Hormone Boost* doesn't start with a detox, which would naturally remove these things from your diet. If you're looking for a detox, all the information you need can be found in *The Supercharged Hormone Diet,* or you can download my New Year Detox, Step 1–30-Day Digestive and Yeast Cleanse from shop.drnatashaturner.com.

Supplement Suggestions

- **Make sure you include the foundation supplements of the Hormone Boost** (explained in Part Three) in your daily regimen. Vitamin E, probiotics and magnesium are particularly important.

- **Clear Detox – Hormonal Health:** I highly recommend this for all signs of estrogen imbalance, such as PMS, hot flashes, mood swings, weight gain, belly fat, cravings and low energy. You may take this for one month or even one year, as it is safe for long-term use.

- **A special note on omega oils in menopause:** I suggest Pure Form Omega (a plant-based omega supplement) for menopausal women because it contains flax and evening primrose oils, which help with the symptoms of hormonal imbalance. This formula is particularly helpful for skin and artery health. I recently called this product "brain food" in a social media post, because I've noticed my memory and recall are much better while I'm taking it. What's more, a colleague, Dr. Jeff Matheson, recently contacted me to share news of a case of mild dementia he observed to improve dramatically after just six weeks of taking the Pure Form supplement. Take two to three capsules twice daily.

- **For the treatment of menopausal symptoms (specifically low estrogen), use phytoestrogenic herbs:** The best options include black cohosh, angelica, red clover extract, sage and licorice, all of which can be used to support healthy estrogen balance.
  - > *Black cohosh* can be used to treat hot flashes, night sweats, vaginal dryness, urinary urgency and other symptoms that can occur during menopause. Take 40 mg twice daily, away from food.

> *Angelica* has been used for ages to treat many symptoms of menopause (hot flashes, etc.), lack of menstrual cycle (amenorrhea) and PMS. It is anti-inflammatory and may help to relieve menstrual cramps because of its anti-spasmodic properties. Take 400 mg one to three times a day, away from food.

> *Red clover* contains high quantities of plant-based estrogens called isoflavones, which may improve menopausal symptoms, reduce the risk of bone loss and lower the risk of heart disease by improving blood pressure and increasing HDL cholesterol. Research on the effectiveness of red clover for the treatment of menopause has, however, yielded conflicting evidence; some reports show it is beneficial, while others claim it is no more helpful than a placebo. You can try taking 80 mg of red clover each day to see if it does the trick for you. Look for Promensil, which appears to be the most extensively researched product.

> *Sage* is an excellent choice to support healthy estrogen balance, especially if sweating and hot flashes are your predominant menopausal symptoms. Take 400 mg once a day, away from food.

> *Licorice* has phytoestogenic properties and is an especially great choice if you're feeling burned out or stressed. Take 300 to 900 mg a day before 3 p.m. Because licorice is stimulating, it should not be taken later in the day and should be avoided completely if you have high blood pressure.

> *Complete your prescription for estrogen balance with Clear Estrogen:* Sometimes a blend of estrogenic herbs is what works best. This formula contains most of the herbs listed above. Take two to four capsules daily, but decrease the dosage if you experience breast pain or swelling. This

product is only herbal, but it is potent and works remarkably well for menopausal symptoms.

- **For PMS or low progesterone, consider Clear Progesterone:** This formula contains a combination of progesterone-supporting herbs and others that support optimal progesterone function. One main ingredient is chasteberry extract (vitex), which increases progesterone by stimulating the production of luteinizing hormone. Take one to four capsules per day of Clear Progesterone, or you can take chasteberry (200 to 300 mg per day, away from food) on its own. Regardless of your choice of product, you should continue the use of the herb(s) for at least three to six months.
- **If you are menopausal or the stressed-out PMS type, take melatonin:** It enhances sex hormone balance, improves sleep and aids weight loss! I recommend 3 to 6 mg per night. Clear Balance – Stress Support also helps with hot flashes and stress symptoms, at any age.

Men, I haven't forgotten about you. Check out my suggestions for a testosterone boost in Chapter 3 and consider implementing them in your daily routine.

Lifestyle Suggestions

Many of the following recommendations are discussed at various points in *The Hormone Boost*, but here are a few extras.

- Do regular aerobic, strengthening and weight-bearing exercise. Aim for 3.5 hours a week.
- Maintain your ideal body weight.
- Stop smoking.
- Use a natural lubricant for vaginal dryness (like Hathor Aphrodisia Lubricant), and speak to your doctor about a prescription for compounded vaginal estriol suppositories. One

to 2 mg inserted once per night for seven nights, and then one to three times per week, ongoing, to eliminate vaginal dryness in just weeks and help maintain bladder health. And remember: use it or lose it! The composition of vaginal walls changes without sexual activity. Vaginal dryness is an unnecessary and totally treatable condition that could stop you from maintaining this part of your healthy lifestyle!

- Utilize stress-management techniques such as breathing exercises, yoga or relaxation response exercises.
- Have regular annual physical exams. I highly recommend a breast ultrasound (I am a fan of this test, combined with a breast MRI if necessary, for breast health more than of a mammogram) and pelvic ultrasound.
- Request bone mineral density testing if you are concerned about osteoporosis.
- Request a blood lipid panel at least yearly. And make sure your TSH stays in the optimal range (head back to Chapter 1 for a refresher on this topic).

Step Four: Protect Your Skin Barrier

The last of the four simple steps for your body is an interesting one that focuses on your largest organ: your skin (according to *National Geographic*, the average adult has 22 square feet—amazing!). Just a few years ago, learning the importance of the skin barrier as a new aspect of hormonal health—and particularly of potential hormone disruption—was an exciting discovery for me. Your skin plays a key role as the protector and gatekeeper of your body, which helps to explain the term "skin barrier," the protectant between the outside world and the human body. And while your skin keeps you looking your best, the latest research shows it's time to examine the toxins entering our body from the outside and to pay attention to our skin barrier.

Skin is the mirror of overall health that:

- prevents bacteria and viruses from entering the body
- protects internal organs, muscles, nerves and blood vessels
- produces melanin to filter harmful UV rays
- metabolizes and activates vitamin D_3 when exposed to the sun
- regulates core body temperature
- excretes excess salt and waste
- retains fluids and moisture, protecting against dehydration
- communicates sensations such as pain, touch, pressure and temperature
- increases surface friction to facilitate basic motor tasks such as grasping, rubbing and scratching
- impacts psychological well-being, because it portrays a specific image of health and well-being to the outside world

Neuropeptides, the chemicals released by the skin's nerve endings, are the skin's first line of defense against infection and trauma. When responding to protect the skin, neuropeptides can create inflammation and uncomfortable skin sensations, such as numbness, itching or tingling. Neuropeptides are nasty creatures that we once assumed stayed within the skin. Recent findings have revealed, though, that they work their way into our brains and increase stress, directly affecting our emotions. For example, finding a pimple on your big date night and becoming stressed out can aggravate your emotional state of being, which in turn can flare up other skin areas. The American Academy of Dermatology explains that the outer layer of our skin can be compromised simply by stress. And since our skin acts as a barrier between us and the outside world, it's important to de-stress as much as possible. Our skin craves moisture, so adding some quenching to our daily skin regimen can be a great way to overcome the irritations and bacteria that can cause larger skin problems down the road.

Of course, we all know the benefits of developing "thick skin." The media, with its advertisements for celebrity-branded creams and bottles that promise miracle results, are constantly reminding us how fragile our skin is. However, anyone suffering from an inflammatory skin condition such as eczema or acne knows that not all skin creams can prevent the boatload of stress on our bodies and its resulting negative effects. When stress pumps through our system, unwanted hormones like cortisol surge, creating an excess that directly leads to more weight gain. Top this with the effect these hormones have on our immune system, speeding up the aging process, and it's little wonder our expensive creams aren't working! It's a catch-22; the initial damage only fuels more skin barrier damage and an increase of cortisol, which keeps the cycle going.

The best defense is a good offense—prevent the problem in the first place. But we often do things that unintentionally damage the skin barrier, such as:

- Go out unprotected in the sun
- Wash with water that is too cold or too hot
- Use harsh cleansers that strip moisture from our skin, or harsh scrubs that can tear the skin's surface
- Soak in water until skin "prunes," which is a sign of barrier damage
- Use skin-care products that contain irritating ingredients like sodium lauryl sulphate, parabens or alcohol
- Over-exfoliate with products that contain high amounts of active ingredients such as alpha-hydroxy acid, beta hydroxy acid or vitamin A (retinol) or use drying anti-acne medications.

What's more, a study published in the *Journal of Investigative Dermatology* (June 2009) confirmed that there is a link between the skin barrier's role and food allergies. The cause of true food allergies—the kind that produce severe or anaphylactic reactions—involves IgE antibodies in the immune system, while food *intolerances* can arise when we consume the same foods day after day with little variety; these are IgG antibody mediated. This dietary stagnation causes the body to become "sensitized" to a particular food. Food intolerances are less intense and typically appear not immediately but rather within 12 to 48 hours after eating the offending food. In my practice, skin conditions such as acne, eczema and psoriasis are commonly connected to food intolerances, and they are greatly reduced when the key culprits are removed and the proper topical products to improve skin barrier health are used.

The evidence supporting the connection between the skin barrier and food allergies continues to grow. A study published in the *Journal of Investigative Dermatology* (July 2013) included more than 600 infants who were three months old and exclusively breastfed from birth. They were tested for eczema and checked to see if they were sensitized to the six most common allergenic foods—wheat, corn, dairy, soy, citrus and gluten. It's believed that the breakdown of the skin barrier in infants with eczema leaves the skin's active immune cells exposed to environmental allergens—in this case, food proteins—which then triggers an allergic immune response. *So not only do food allergies cause eczema, eczema causes food allergies.* That's a hard situation to be in, but it's one you can resolve.

Do-It-Yourself Beauty

One of the best ways to ensure that your skin-care products contain no harmful toxins or additives is to make them yourself. A few hours of research on reliable websites combined with a quick shopping trip for the organic ingredients, and you can be making your own facial cleanser (raw honey and coconut oil), facial serum (rosehip seed oil plus a combination of essential oils) and body moisturizer (jojoba oil, coconut oil, shea butter, cocoa butter and essential oils). You're in control of the amounts and expense, and, after a bit of practice (read: some inevitable failures before real success), your skin will be the envy of your friends.

Nutrition

It's no surprise that diet can play a large role in building a strong skin barrier. To get to the bottom of your symptoms, I recommend a 14-day elimination diet to remove the most common food allergens from your diet. This will give your body a break, alleviate immune-system stress and provide an overall detox. Slowly reintroducing each food can allow you to connect particular symptoms with your food choices. This is the same diet approach I mentioned earlier, in the simple step to optimize your digestion. It is laid out for you, including recipes and permitted food lists, in *The Supercharged Hormone Diet*. If you don't want to do a 14-day elimination diet, blood IgG food allergy testing is also an option.

Stress Management

Once you get rid of food allergies, make sure you follow the sleep tips, diet rules and stress-busters discussed throughout this book. During times of stress or anxiety, skin inflammation increases as a way to protect the skin from harm. So if you already have inflammation in your skin, as with eczema, stress will worsen your condition. The cortisol increase associated with chronic stress can also suppress the effectiveness of the immune system. Your epidermal skin cells lie on top of each other and are tightly packed together, forming a strong barrier that blocks the penetration of bacteria and other pathogens. When you are under stress, however, this protective outermost layer of skin becomes impaired. In one study, researchers examined the skin of 27 students in three situations: just after returning from winter vacation (low stress), during final exams (high stress) and during spring break (low stress). Their findings demonstrate that stress caused the outermost layer of skin to break up as skin cells shrank and the lipids between these cells evaporated. These tiny cracks make the skin more permeable, allowing harmful bacteria to infiltrate the deeper layers of skin. The bacteria produce a protein that activates the immune system, leading to outbreaks of eczema and psoriasis and increasing acne inflammation.

Supplements

Consider your skin-care selections, including your moisturizer, as topical supplements for your skin. Be sure to apply after showering and before bed to protect and maintain your skin barrier. A product like those in the Biophora skin-care line, or something offering similar ingredients, is a good choice (You can visit my website to purchase these skin-care products.) The Biophora system has been created in collaboration with cosmetic plastic surgeons, anti-aging specialists, naturopathic doctors and chemists. These state-of-the-art products and protocols are designed to make skin science understandable and skin maintenance simple for you.

After treating your skin with the right stuff on the outside, it's time to work on the inside. The foundation supplements described in Chapter 11 are perfect for boosting skin health *and* the activity of the six fat-loss hormones. This is especially true for vitamin C, vitamin E, probiotics and essential fatty acid supplements like Pure Form Omega.

We've detoxed the kitchen, bathroom and bedroom. We've optimized digestion and given our liver some much-needed love. Throw in some sex, massage, meditation and laughter—not to mention attending to our skin barrier—and we've walked through the simple steps toward optimal hormonal health. Now you're ready to start the Hormone Boost nutrition, supplement and exercise plans.

THE CLIENT: Elizabeth R.

DETAILS: Female, 61

**BODY COMPOSITION RESULTS (FROM SCALE AND BODY FAT/
MUSCLE MASS VIA BIO-IMPEDANCE TESTING)**

MEASUREMENT	BEFORE	AFTER	TOTAL LOSS/GAIN
Weight (lb.)	185	142	(-) 43
Lean Body Mass (lb.)	118.2	113.7	(-) 4.5
Fat Mass (lb.)	66.8	28.3	(-) 38.5
Basal Metabolic Rate (calories/day)	1,679 calories	1,559 calories	(-) 120

This lady is one of my coolest patients. She's hip, motivated, super health-conscious and so fun to work with. During the span of just under one year, from October 2014 to October 2015, she lost almost 40 pounds of fat! In addition to the fat loss, her energy, sleep, strength, vitality and menopausal symptoms all improved.

Elizabeth's case is a perfect example of what an unbalanced carb-rich, protein-deficient vegan diet can do. She had gained over 30 pounds trying to be vegan and it backfired with her metabolism, as it will with most if special effort is not paid to ensure adequate protein intake and carb-consciousness.

PART THREE

THE HORMONE BOOST ACTION PLAN

*Good things come to people who wait, but better
things come to those who go out and get them.*

ANONYMOUS

CHAPTER 10

THE HORMONE BOOST
NUTRITION PLAN

In the end, it's not the years in your life
that count. It's the life in your years.

ABRAHAM LINCOLN

Welcome! You have reached the place where your prep work is done and the action plan begins. If weight loss is one of your health goals at this stage, you can start by avoiding a common mistake that so many of us make: If we recognize that our weight is not coming off, we start eating less. I know this all too well. My struggle with hormonal imbalance and thyroid disease began after graduation from university years ago, when I gained over 25 pounds—despite exercising an hour a day and counting every calorie. The harder I strived, the more I failed.

Now I know why—when we cut calories drastically, we cause stress on our bodies, which increases our cortisol, which sabotages all our efforts. This stress hormone causes our appetite for comfort foods to surge, is associated with belly fat (even in people who are otherwise thin) and slows down our metabolism by suppressing our thyroid hormone.

You can restore hormone balance *and* lose weight by *eating the right foods at the right times in the right combinations* to optimize your fat-burning hormones. This, plus *moderate* exercise, is the secret to success. The rules in this chapter are built upon the principles of my original Hormone Diet plan; the basic foundation of eating the right foods at the right times, and avoiding the wrong foods 80 to 100 percent of the time, still applies.

The Right Foods

Healthy eating is not about strict dietary limitations, staying unrealistically thin or depriving yourself of the foods you love. Rather, it's about feeling great, having more energy, improving your outlook and stabilizing your mood. And the right foods power up the hormones that do just that. Eat properly and you can increase metabolism, energy, mood and your brain power. Here's how:

- **Eat lean protein, low-glycemic carbohydrates, fiber and healthy fats at each meal.** This approach keeps your blood sugar stable and your energy up and boosts the glucagon that burns fat (it also works in opposition to insulin, which signals the body to store fat and increases appetite and cravings). Adding fiber to each meal also increases adiponectin. Taking in a steady supply of protein throughout the day is also important, because it boosts the hormones that help us burn fat (glucagon) and those that control our appetite and make us feel full (like peptide YY in the gut), *every time we eat it.* Furthermore, essential amino acids—the building blocks of protein necessary to produce thyroid hormone, serotonin, dopamine, melatonin and growth hormone— cannot be manufactured by the body, so they *must* be a vital component of our diet.
- **Calculate your specific daily guidelines for protein intake,** which includes the range between the minimum amount needed to preserve your muscle mass and the ideal amount you should consume to encourage muscle growth. You have

a daily range of 1.6 to 2.2 g of protein per kilogram of body weight. On the days you strength-train and do yoga, you need to consume protein based on the 2.2 g calculation. On other days, you should not go below a minimum amount of protein, calculated at 1.6 g per kilogram. (To calculate your protein intake range, take your weight in pounds and divide it by 2.2 to find your weight in kilograms, then multiply this amount by 1.6 and 2.2 to find your daily range of protein intake.) I recommend sticking to your calculated minimum if you have more than 40 pounds to lose. In the meal plans outlined in Part Four, you'll see that the recommended protein servings range from 25 to 35 g per meal, which will hit an average-sized person's needs, but you are free to tweak the recipes once you've done your own calculation. You can choose to consume your protein divided among (a) three meals plus one dose of protein closer to bedtime, if needed (e.g., one serving of whey protein powder mixed with one serving of Clear Recovery), (b) four meals or (c) two meals plus two shakes (from smoothie recipes or a meal replacement like Clear Complete). Whatever works for you on a given day with your schedule works for me too.

- **Avoid starchy carbs at breakfast.** Sticking to a high-protein breakfast increases thyroid hormone and sets your dopamine levels for the day—which means you will enjoy better appetite control and be craving-free while also avoiding that mid-afternoon slump. This means breads, cereals, bagels, etc., are off limits. The first few days may feel challenging, but I promise it will quickly become second nature. You can choose any meal option from Part Four that is free of starchy carbs; I have even included fruit-free smoothie recipes if you want to skip fruit as a carb source at breakfast too.
- **Choose a completely carb-free breakfast to kick your fat-burning plan into high gear.** Skipping fruit and other carbs

at breakfast helps to keep you in the same ketogenic (fat-burning) state that happens overnight, and which lasts until your first carb-containing meal of the day. I don't usually recommend this right away—I like to save it as a tweak for later use. You may want to kick in the carb-free breakfast as a means of tricking your metabolism, though, if you feel your results are slowing down or if you've hit a weight-loss plateau.

- **Ditch snacking.** After almost 17 years of clinical practice and three bestselling books, I have seen a number of similar trends over and over. A big one is the mid-afternoon snack that seems to lack sufficient protein and offers too many carbs and too much fat. To escape this dieting mistake, the Hormone Boost plan ditches the snacks. Instead you will eat three or four equal-sized meals and avoid sabotaging your results by failing to consume enough protein. We've been hearing about the importance of eating three square meals a day for years, and the advice might not be as outdated as it seems. If you consume enough protein, avoid excess carbs at mealtimes and eat regularly, you can avoid messing with the hormones that keep weight off. But if you skip meals, wait too long between meals, fail to consume enough protein, or eat the wrong foods, your body will experience more dips and spikes than it should—and that will throw your hormones, such as insulin and cortisol, out of whack. Specifically, waiting too long to eat between meals causes a blood sugar drop, which triggers a stress response in your body, which in turn releases cortisol—and causes your energy to crash hard. This causes you to overeat at your next meal, leading to a blood sugar and insulin spike. You can break this cycle by eating three or four square meals. If you choose to eat four times a day, have a meal that contains whey protein as your third one, to cut cravings and balance cortisol so you will eat less at your next meal. Many of my patients like to eat four times per day, as do I, so the meal plan outlined in Part Four is based on four meals, but you can tweak any recipe to suit your protein needs if you choose to eat three or five times per day.

- **Have your starchy carb after 4 p.m., as part of your evening meal.** The concept of eating your carbs early in the day because you will have a better chance of burning them off could actually be setting you up for cravings all day long. Eating a starchy carb—like potatoes or beans—early in the day creates cravings for them later. So I suggest you eat only one, with your last meal. Do not combine your starchy carb selection with fruit in your evening meal. Chose one or the other, not both. At this point in the day, that carb will raise your serotonin levels, which helps with sleep. And sleep is one of the best fat-burning activities when we create the optimum conditions for it, as laid out in Chapter 8. Consuming at least one starchy carb per day also helps to maintain testosterone. A diet free of starchy carbs lowers testosterone and serotonin and increases stress hormones. Last, don't forget the impact that eating starch only with the evening meal has on boosting adiponectin during the day: this can lead to greater weight loss and seems to be easier to do than restrict carbs at night. And we all know that any diet you stick to is the one for you.

- **Do the Hormone Boost cleanse day.** Studies have clearly shown that our bodies respond to fasting by boosting glucagon, adiponectin and growth hormone—the hormone that helps build muscle. Intermittent fasting involves avoiding food intake for one day per week. During your cleanse day, you should *drink at least four quarts of warm or cold herbal teas* to support the cleansing process. I recommend a combination of herbs with anti-inflammatory and diuretic effects, such as ginger, lemon, blueberry, hibiscus, dandelion, green tea and parsley. Alternatively, you can use an intermittent fasting support like Clear Cleanse, mixed into four quarts of water to drink throughout the day. If you feel overly hungry, you can consume one or two hard-boiled eggs in the morning or a serving of nuts in the afternoon, but try to last the day. You can also try your cleanse day by first consuming breakfast and then embarking on the cleansing drinks for the next 24 hours. The benefits of fasting extend beyond just the 24 hours, and it does get easier with time and experience. You can do this once every 7 to 10 days, or even more than once a week if you want to accelerate your plan. I recommend doing your cleanse days have on Tuesdays or Wednesdays. If you have your cheat meal (see next page) on the weekend, as so many of us do, this will give you a day or two of clean eating to get your insulin back in balance, quiet cravings and steady your appetite. I actually spoke about this tip on an episode of the *Dr. Oz Show* (Google "hump day cleanse Dr. Oz," and you should be able to find the clip).

- **Avoid hormone-hindering foods 100 percent of the time.** This means you should *never* consume the following products:
  - > Processed meats and luncheon meats: Instead, visit your local deli or butcher and ask for preservative-free (nitrate-free) sliced meats.
  - > Fructose-sweetened foods or foods containing high-fructose corn syrup (HFCS): HFCS increases appetite and cravings.
  - > Foods containing aspartame or other artificial sweeteners, which raise insulin and contribute to cravings and weight gain.
  - > Agave and limit stevia: Avoid agave and limit intake of stevia to a maximum of once a day. I have seen excessive consumption of canned drinks or protein bars sweetened with stevia slow weight loss in some patients.
  - > Farmed salmon: A 2004 study found higher toxin levels in farmed salmon than in wild-caught.

> Foods containing artificial coloring, preservatives, sulfites and nitrates.
> Trans fatty acids (any hydrogenated oils, partially hydrogenated oils, shortenings, margarines) and unhealthy processed (like sunflower and safflower) inflammatory fats (including cottonseed oil, palm oil and products labeled as vegetable oil).
> Peanuts, unless they are organic and, optimally, aflatoxin-free.

- **Have a cheat meal once a week.** Your only restriction is that you must not consume any of the foods you are to avoid 100 percent of the time (see the list in the previous bullet point); otherwise anything is fair game. Why the cheat meal? Continuous extreme caloric restriction is not an effective long-term fat-loss solution; it is simply not sustainable. The short-term victories achieved with that type of eating are *always* followed with rebound weight gain because, whether we like it or not, hormones will kick in to return the body to its status quo. From a physiological standpoint, a cheat meal serves to increase your thyroid hormone (particularly the conversion of T4 to T3), lower levels of reverse T3 (which can block the action of T3) and generally boost your metabolism. Remember that the human body is an adaptive machine— when you reduce overall calories, the body adapts and lowers your metabolism as a survival mechanism. Believe it or not, introducing a weekly cheat meal keeps your metabolism guessing and actually increases your long-term success. It prevents hunger and cravings and refuels your muscles' energy stores, particularly glycogen, which helps to maintain strength and endurance for your workouts. I usually advise my patients to begin incorporating their cheat meal after two weeks on the Hormone Boost plan. Note: If your weight is up two to three days after a cheat meal, you have overdone your cheat meal. Here are the foods you should avoid 80 percent of the time—so restrict these to a maximum of one serving a week, during your cheat meal:

> White flour, enriched flour, refined flour, wheat flour, white sugar, white potatoes and white rice
> Saturated fats in full-fat dairy products and red meat
> Large fish known to be high in mercury, including swordfish, shark, tilefish, marlin, orange roughy, grouper, king mackerel and tuna
> Raisins, figs and dates, which are high in sugar

• **Go for the Hormone Boost foods.** There are certain foods with additional hormone boost properties that you may want to include in your diet. I have touched on them at various points in this book and will do so again later in this chapter, but here's a quick list of them:

> Nuts, especially walnuts, as a fat source.
> Pears—think of them as the new apple. Have them a few times a week as your carb selection at a meal.
> Low-fat cheese is a protein source to have at least once daily, if you can tolerate dairy. (It is listed in the protein section of the Foods to Enjoy in Part Four.)
> Whey protein should be the protein source for your 4 p.m. meal (options include ricotta cheese, whey protein powder, Greek yogurt Clear Complete meal replacement, and protein bars with whey protein base, such as the B-UP bar).
> Olive oil or hemp hearts are my favorite option for your fat at breakfast. Olive oil boosts adiponectin and shrinks the size of your fat cells. Hemp hearts provide a rich source of GLA oil, which is great for combating belly fat, reducing inflammation and moisturizing your skin.
> Tomato juice—I always go for this option on flights—with water to combat sodium. Although it may sound like

strange advice, the natural acidic quality of this tasty drink offers us weight-loss benefits, and because it boosts adiponectin when consumed once a day, it can reduce belly fat. Drinking something acidic after your meal is known to reduce the glycemic load (or blood sugar impact), which then blunts the increase of insulin and leads to less sugar being stored as fat.

> Go blue when your carb source in a meal comes from fruit. Adiponectin is naturally released when we exercise. Produced by our fat cells, it increases metabolism, improves insulin sensitivity and reduces inflammation and the risk of heart disease. It appears that blueberries are the only fruit to stimulate the release of this hormone—thanks to a phytonutrient found in blueberries' skin. Additionally, blueberries help fat loss by improving insulin balance. A recent study showed that obese people who drank one blueberry smoothie a day for six weeks had a 22 percent improvement in insulin sensitivity, which ultimately equates to better fat metabolism. Just a half a cup per day will do the trick.

- **Eat fresh, locally grown organic produce** and, whenever you can, choose organic or wild sources of meat, fish, eggs and dairy, which are free of hormone-disrupting additives, hormones and pesticides.
- **Drink two cups of water before each meal.** Studies have shown that those who follow this habit lose more weight in 12 weeks than those who do not.
- **Pay attention to your cravings.** If your diet is hormonally balanced, you should be craving-free. An out-of-control appetite or desire for something sweet, however, usually means you are not consuming enough protein, are taking in too much carbohydrate or are sleep deprived or stressed out.

The Hormone Boost is all about boosting your fat loss, strength and energy. According to a 2011 study published in Vienna's *Wiener Medizinische Wochenschrift*, nutrition plays a hugely important role in the prevention of sarcopenia (loss of muscle and increased fragility with age). This will not come as a news flash to Hormone Diet alumni, but I am sharing these results here because they are a great reminder of the associations between several nutritional factors and muscle mass, strength, function and physical performance. Adequate amounts of high-quality protein are integral for the optimal stimulation of muscle protein synthesis. But the study also found that vitamin D, antioxidants (vitamins C and E) and omega-3 polyunsaturated fatty acids may also contribute to the preservation of muscle function. These last three need to be obtained through the foundation portion of the Hormone Boost supplement plan (in Chapter 11). The 2011 study also addressed the importance of physical activity, specifically resistance training, not only to facilitate muscle protein anabolism but also to increase energy expenditure (i.e., metabolism and physical energy), appetite and food intake in elderly people at risk of malnutrition. The Hormone Boost is the plan you need to stay strong and mobile!

The Right Times

Creating the optimal Hormone Boost also requires you to pay attention to *when* you eat. It is impossible to balance your hormones if you skip meals, eat too close to bedtime or have irregular eating habits. These are the simple timing rules you need to follow:

- **Aim to eat about every four hours**. Remember that the thermic effect of food can increase your metabolic rate from 5 to 15 percent after a meal, so not skipping meals and not having only one or two large meals makes for a faster metabolism and better brain power.
- **Enjoy your meals at the same time every day.** People who eat at the same times daily have lower blood sugar and insulin levels, which fosters better hormonal balance for fat loss.

- **Eat within an hour of rising and try to avoid eating within the three-hour period before bedtime.** Breaking your overnight fast with protein boosts thyroid hormone and ignites your metabolism for the day, while eating too close to bedtime raises your body temperature and interferes with the natural fat-burning effects of sleep, by reducing melatonin and growth hormone. The exception is a dose of protein and amino acids close to bedtime, which can help to preserve muscle tissue and support fat loss during sleep. (If you wish, you can consume a bit of protein mixed with branched-chain amino acids closer to bedtime, like $^1/_2$ scoop of Clear Recovery and $^1/_2$ to 1 scoop of Dream Protein mixed in water.)
- **If you consume alcohol with your meal, enjoy it *after* you eat to enhance the hormones involved in digestion and appetite control.** But that also means you need to skip the starch with your meal (such as quinoa), or you will end up consuming too much carbohydrate at one sitting.
- **Always eat within 45 minutes of finishing your workout.** This meal or snack should not contain much fat and should be higher in carbohydrate, with a bit of protein. This combination will maximize the release of growth hormone and stimulate muscle repair and building. I suggest liquid protein meals post-workout, such as a smoothie or a protein-rich recovery drink. This will provide readily available protein for muscle growth and repair. In fact, MariaLisa, one of the success stories shared in this book, increased her muscle mass over a three-month period simply by adopting this practice.
- **For optimal strength and performance, never do your weight training on an empty stomach.** You need adequate food to ensure that you have enough energy to get through your workout effectively. You may complete your cardio training before eating, however, if your session is 30 minutes or less.

Your Daily Meal Schedule

Here's a look at how your daily meal schedule might shape up during your Hormone Boost. Note that this is just an overview of a typical day and that you can tweak the plan to suit your specific needs. To ensure that every day is a success on the Hormone Boost plan, I have included a number of recipes in Part Four. The recipes are divided into meals containing a starchy carb (suitable for meal 4) and meals free of a starchy carb (suitable for meals 1, 2 and 3).

You will follow this schedule most days of the week—with a cheat meal once a week and a Hormone Boost intermittent fasting day once every 7 to 10 days.

7–8 a.m.: A Brain, Metabolic and Energy Boost

You'll start your day with a breakfast that contains at least 30 g of protein, which will ignite your metabolism (thyroid hormone) for the day. The Hormone Boost avoids starchy carbs at breakfast, to control your blood sugar for the day and prevent cravings. This also helps to improve mental function and focus, because it sets your dopamine status for the day. A sample meal choice would be an omelet with two or three eggs and goat cheese served with an optional side of mixed greens such as arugula and baby spinach, topped with toasted pumpkin and sesame seeds with Celtic sea salt. Sprinkle ground flax or chia on the meal to increase the fiber content. You can enjoy one cup of organic coffee—with cream and cinnamon—for a dopamine boost.

11 a.m.–1 p.m.: An Energy and Metabolic Boost

The second meal keeps your metabolic engines running, your blood sugars balanced and your energy high with the right combination of macronutrients. You want to boost blood sugar for energy—but not too much! A sample meal choice would be sliced turkey, feta, strawberries and Vidalia onion on a bed of greens, topped with toasted pine nuts or pumpkin seeds. Toss on some chia to increase your fiber intake.

3–4 p.m.: An Energy and Cortisol-Balancing Boost
Regular mealtimes and consistency are vital to help stress recovery, fat-burning and unbalanced sugars. This is also the time of day to include certain foods known to improve adrenal gland health, like a source of whey protein, to avoid the 3 to 4 p.m. crash, as well as to keep from overeating in the evening. A sample meal choice would be a shake made with one serving of whey protein powder, 1 tablespoon of almond butter or walnut butter, one serving of a fiber supplement and almond milk, cashew milk or water.

6–7 p.m.: A Fat-Burning, Mood and Sleep Repair Boost
Now is the time to think of boosting the hormones that help your mood (serotonin) and prepare for nighttime rejuvenation (melatonin and growth hormone). In order to achieve this goal, meal 4 is the only meal of the day that contains a starchy carb selection. A sample meal choice would be $^1/_2$ cup of quinoa (your best low-carb grain option) topped with a tasty chicken curry stir-fry.

Now that you have a clear sense of the *right foods* and the *right timing*, you can use the food lists in Part Four to create the *right combinations*: your own Hormone Boost meals, smoothies and salads. All you need to do is select one protein, one carb, one fat and one fiber four times a day—keeping in mind which carbs can be consumed at which time of day. Your grocery shopping list for the whole diet as well as smoothies is also in Part Four.

Grocery Shopping on the Hormone Boost Plan
Ensuring that you have the right foods on hand at all times is important. It makes everything a whole lot easier—you can't cook what's missing, or eat what's not around! While you shop, understanding

nutrition labels and the glycemic index will help you find Hormone Boost options. Just follow these guidelines on how to read nutrition labels carefully:

- **Start with the ingredients.** If the product contains any of the hormone-hindering ingredients that you are to avoid 100 percent of the time, put it back on the shelf. Don't be afraid to write these on a piece of paper or type them into your phone. It's better to have this information on hand and make the right choices than to rely on a memory that hasn't yet been boosted.

- **Move on to the nutrition label and check the serving size.** A serving size of five potato chips doesn't make much sense based on the amount most of us would really eat in a sitting. Sometimes foods look as though they are a good choice for you, but only because the serving size used to report the nutrition values is completely unrealistic.

- **Check the amount of carbohydrate.** Read the amount listed on the label and compare it with the total amount of carbohydrate you should consume per meal and snack, which is in the chart on page 199 (these are the only numbers you will need to memorize, I promise!). If the product's carbohydrate content per serving is higher than the amount in the chart, look for something else. I also want you to compare the amount of carbohydrate relative to protein.

- **Check the amount of protein.** Remember this simple guideline: If the product contains similar amounts of protein and carbohydrate or, even better, more protein than carbs per serving, it is a good choice for you. For example, vanilla soy milk has 11 g of carbs and 6 g of protein; plain soy milk has 3 g of carbs and 6 g of protein. In this case, plain soy milk is a much better choice.

- **Check the fat content.** Compare it to the total amount of fat you should consume in a meal or snack (again, noted in the chart below). Check the saturated fat content in particular and aim for little to none, but certainly no more than 3 g per serving. Here's another guideline for hormonal health: *High protein supersedes low fat.* So, if you have to decide between a product that has more protein but also slightly more fat over another that has lower protein as well as lower fat, I suggest that you still go for the higher protein option.

- **Check the fiber content.** Products that contain less than 2 g of fiber per serving are not great choices. If you have a number of brands to choose from, select the product that's highest in fiber (and, if possible, also lowest in carbs and highest in protein).
- **Check the sodium content.** Products with less than 140 mg of salt are considered low-sodium options. Remember, you should consume only 2,300 mg of sodium per day, which is equal to about a teaspoon of table salt. When comparing products, pick the one that's lowest in sodium. Sometimes I may end up consuming more sodium if the product happens to have a great protein and carb balance. Just remember to keep up your water intake, and avoid high-sodium options completely if you have high blood pressure.
- **Don't waste time checking the calorie count.** It's really not necessary; any food that is too high in carb or fat, and therefore high in calories, will be avoided by following these label-reading guidelines.

WOMEN: NUTRITIONAL GUIDELINES PER MEAL	MEN: NUTRITIONAL GUIDELINES PER MEAL
Protein: 25–35 g	Protein: 35–45 g
Carbs: 20–30 g	Carbs: 30–40 g
Fats: 10–14 g	Fats: 14–18 g
Fiber: 4–10 g	Fiber: 4–10 g

The "Greatest Hits"

Before we leave the topic of food and move on to supplements and exercise, I want to share with you several powerful food-related hints and tips that really stand out for me as being worth extra attention. The foods featured in this section are like hormonal "greatest hits." At first glance, they appear to lend weight to the existence of certain superfoods—certainly, the nutrients they contain have been shown to have several health-promoting properties. If you haven't yet included these foods in your diet, I hope this summary motivates you to seek them out and follow these simple nutrition tips.

Power Up Your Brain with Greens

Adding more spinach, kale, collards and mustard greens to your diet could help slow cognitive decline and keep your mental abilities sharp, according to new research published by the Federation of American Societies for Experimental Biology (March 2015). The study also examined the nutrients responsible for the effect, linking vitamin K consumption to slower cognitive decline for the first time. Top off at least one or two of your meals daily with 2 cups of greens.

Blueberries Are the Best!

Maintaining your mood for optimal daytime energy goes beyond how much sleep you've had. So do a daily mental check—if you have signs of worry, dwelling, obsessing, sleep disruption or carb cravings, your serotonin could use a boost.

Blueberries could be just the trick. As a 2015 press release from the American Physiological Society notes, this fruit shows promise as a mood elevator, perhaps even as treatment for post-traumatic stress disorder (PTSD). Researchers at Louisiana State University discovered that blueberries can regulate neurotransmitter levels, which in turn can increase the ability of SSRIs (the only approved therapy for PTSD) to increase serotonin levels.

But that's not all—the journal *Molecular Nutrition & Food Research*

(2013) notes that blueberries also contain pterostilbene, a compound that works with vitamin D to boost immune function. A clinical trial presented at the meeting of the American Heart Association in 2012 found that pterostilbene additionally reduces blood pressure, while researchers working with the Spanish Biomedical Research Center discovered that pterostilbene also lowers the accumulation of body fat (*Journal of Agricultural and Food Chemistry* 2014).

Go for the bluest: The blue in blueberries signals the presence of anthocyanins—a powerful group of antioxidants. In 2014, researchers at South Dakota State University listed the multiple health benefits of blueberries, including improved brain and nervous system function, as well as benefits for the eyes and urinary tract.

If these aren't reasons enough to make blueberries one of your go-to foods, consider this—their polyphenolics have, according to researchers at the American Chemical Society (2010), antioxidant and anti-inflammatory effects on the brain, that offer protection against memory loss and other age-related mental deficits!

The "Other" Berries: Think Purple

While less familiar than blueberries and cranberries, the "purple berries"—elderberry, black currant and chokeberry—are as much as 50 percent higher in antioxidants than lighter-colored berries, according to research by a group of U.S. Department of Agriculture scientists, published by the *American Chemical Society* in 2004. Make purple berries a regular part of your diet and experience significant health benefits, including protection against cancer, heart disease and Alzheimer's.

Pear is the New Apple to Manage Diabetes

While "an apple a day keeps the doctor away" is a common saying, researchers at North Dakota State University and the University of Massachusetts (2015) discovered that including Starkrimson or Bartlett pears as part of your daily diet can help manage Type 2

**The Best Thing You Can
Do for Your Baby's Health**

We now know how embryos receive vital nutrition during the first 11 weeks of pregnancy, thanks to scientists at Manchester University's Institute of Human Development (2015). Their research also suggests that optimal nutrition *before* conception is important; nutrients stored in the mother's gland cells will be delivered to the placenta after conception and converted into amino acids that enable the embryo's growth during the first trimester. This is a crucial developmental stage for healthy fetuses, and it emphasizes just how essential a healthy diet is for mothers. In other words, all the careful eating choices you make before *and* after conception pay off for your baby!

diabetes and diabetes-induced hypertension. It turns out these refreshing fruits contain phenolic compounds that offer a variety of health benefits, thanks to their antioxidant properties. So reach for a pear, and don't skip the peel—it's got the highest concentration of phenolic content!

The "French Paradox": Maybe It's the Cheese and Not Just the Wine

Among scientists, it's known as the "French paradox"—the French diet is high in saturated fats but the French people have remarkably low cardiovascular disease rates. This seemingly contradictory fact has inspired numerous studies and theories. And the answer to the question why, according to scientists in the *Journal of Agricultural and Food Chemistry* (April 2015), is in your gut.

Although both cheese and butter can share the same fat content, the study found that cheese reduced "bad" cholesterol in a way that butter did not. It turns out that cheese produces butyrate, a compound found in gut bacteria. Elevated butyrate levels appear to reduce cholesterol—which in turn supports a lower incidence of cardiovascular disease in a cheese-consuming population. So, while you wouldn't want to eat cheese with every meal, this research does suggest there's a place for cheese in your diet.

Go Nuts: When What You Eat Affects More Than Your Gut
The U.S. Department of Agriculture's Human Nutrition Research Center released findings (in 2007) suggesting that making walnuts a part of your diet (between 2 and 9 percent of your total food intake) can actually reverse some aspects of aging in the brain.

The alpha-linolenic acid (ALA) in walnuts is an essential omega-3 fatty acid that acts alongside other polyphenols as powerful antioxidants. Together, ALA and polyphenols can block free radicals and their associated inflammation. Eating between 1 and 1.5 ounces of walnuts a day is sufficient to reduce harmful cholesterol, as well as to reduce and delay the onset of age-related mental deficiencies. That's a small handful for a significant brain boost.

A Cup of Tea to Improve Your Memory?
Drinking black or green tea can inhibit the activity of certain enzymes associated with the development of Alzheimer's disease, according to research from Newcastle University published in *Phytotherapy Research* (2004). Both teas diminish the activity of acetylcholinesterase, the enzyme responsible for breaking down the acetylcholine neurotransmitter. A drop in acetylcholine is associated with Alzheimer's disease. If you're choosing between the green and black leaves, think green—it goes one step further and obstructs beta-secretase activity, which also plays a significant role in Alzheimer's disease.

A New Weapon against Heart Disease
If you have abdominal fat, high cholesterol, high blood pressure or abnormal glucose metabolism—all factors that make up metabolic syndrome—you are at risk of heart disease. Because excessive caloric intake is seen as one of the root causes of metabolic syndrome (also known as insulin resistance syndrome), physicians typically prescribe weight loss, exercise and a balanced diet. They could start prescribing Tegreen too, according to research published a decade

ago at an Experimental Biology annual meeting. Tegreen is a tea polyphenols product that contains more than 65 percent tea catechins derived from the leaf. Preliminary studies have shown improved lipid and glucose metabolism, enhanced insulin sensitivity and a balanced metabolic rate of fat deposit and fat burning.

Break Your Fast with Whey

It's now common knowledge that early-morning consumption of certain proteins is good for stimulating the right levels of insulin production. So researchers tested whey protein to see if it too would stimulate the production of glucagon-like peptide-1 (GLP-1)—a gut hormone connected to insulin production—and thus have the potential to improve the body's blood sugar control after eating.

Published in *Diabetologia* (July 2014), this research confirms that whey protein could be an additional tool to help control blood sugar in patients with diabetes. Participants who consumed whey protein before breakfast showed 28 percent lower glucose levels during a 180-minute post-meal period. So if you're trying to manage your blood sugar levels throughout the day, power up with whey. This is also a great trick before your morning strength-training workout. Drink your whey, do your workout and then have your Hormone Boost breakfast (meal 1).

A Spoonful of Safflower Oil

In 2011, *Clinical Research* published study results suggesting that adding a daily dose of safflower oil ($1^2/_3$ teaspoons), a common cooking oil, for 16 weeks can improve good cholesterol, blood sugar, insulin sensitivity and inflammation in certain populations. Participants in the study didn't substitute the safflower oil for any part of their diet, so the reduced abdominal fat and increased muscle tissue results reinforce safflower oil's potential to lower the risk of cardiovascular disease. These benefits appear to be due to the positive effects of safflower oil for boosting our fat-burning friend adiponectin. I recommend four conjugated linoleic acid capsules, such as Clear CLA, as the best daily source of safflower oil.

Your Body on Olive Oil

Olive oil impacts adiponectin activity, according to research results presented in the June 2015 edition of *PLOS One*. This is yet another scientific reason to stick to the good old time-tested Mediterranean diet.

Adiponectin is suppressed in obesity through mechanisms involving chronic inflammation and oxidative stress. Olive oil consumption is associated with beneficial metabolic and cardio-vascular health actions, possibly related to the antioxidant phenol hydroxytyrosol and the monounsaturated fatty acid oleic acid that are naturally present in the oil. Both possess anti-inflammatory and blood vessel protective properties.

Now you know the diet rules and foods that make up your Hormone Boost. The six supplements vital to your success are next.

A HORMONE BOOST REAL-LIFE SUCCESS STORY

THE CLIENT: Anna A.

DETAILS: Female, 49

BODY COMPOSITION RESULTS (FROM SCALE AND BODY FAT/ MUSCLE MASS VIA BIO-IMPEDANCE TESTING)

MEASUREMENT	BEFORE	AFTER	TOTAL LOSS/GAIN
Weight (lb.)	138	130	(-) 8
Lean Body Mass (lb.)	99.3	99.5	(+) 0.2
Fat Mass (lb.)	36.7	27.9	(-) 8.8
Basal Metabolic Rate (calories/day)	1,485 calories	1,504 calories	(+) 19

Anna was one of three women I worked with for six weeks for a special episode of the *Marilyn Denis Show* that was all about losing belly fat—especially the dreaded and stubborn last 10 pounds.

Anna works shifts as a nurse, is in menopause and has hypothyroidism—and a secret addiction to peanut butter cups. Seriously . . . she would eat them in her car! I only met her in person twice—once to give her the supplement, diet and sleeping plans of the Hormone Boost, and the second time six weeks later, to measure her results.

I classified Anna as the "sluggish belly-fat type," because her thyroid, energy and hormones all needed a boost. After six weeks on the program, her sleep and energy were much improved—and she lost six inches around her belly button and nine pounds of fat! (You can watch the show at www.marilyn.ca/mobile/Segment?segid=109608.)

CHAPTER 11

THE HORMONE BOOST
SUPPLEMENT PLAN

I find that the harder I work, the more luck I seem to have.

THOMAS JEFFERSON

Over the past 50 years, our food has grown more and more vitamin deficient. Once upon a time, soils were replete with nutrients, which were transferred into the plants they fed. But as farming techniques have changed dramatically over the past half-century, so has the nutrient content of crops. Fast-forward to today. Many of the foods on our supermarket shelves have been transported, frozen, cooked or processed in ways that strip away much-needed vitamins and minerals. And thanks to our insatiable appetite for foods made with white flour, trans fats and sugar, it's no surprise that few of us are getting the nutrition we need from our daily meals.

Then there are the lifestyle factors. Living with air pollution, drinking coffee, taking medications, consuming alcohol and even exercising—all of these increase our vitamin and mineral requirements. Add various forms of stress to the mixture, and our need for nutrients is higher still. Some sources say our vitamin C is completely sapped after 20 minutes under stress. A deficiency of any nutrient can cause fatigue, poor concentration, malaise, anxiety and increased susceptibility to infections. If left untreated, a nutrient deficiency can eventually lead to a more serious medical condition.

Unless you are ready to leave the city and start growing all your own organic food, the best way to ensure that you're meeting your many vitamin and mineral requirements is through supplementation. Now, taking a raft of supplements every day may not make you feel like turning cartwheels in the street, but you should know that simply taking vitamins C and E daily can reduce your risk of Alzheimer's disease by 58 percent. Is it not worth a little bit of effort now to be sharp and active at 85?

The documented health benefits of multivitamins continue to accumulate. In fact, most major health organizations now recommend the use of a multivitamin daily. Certain nutrients such as vitamin D, folic acid, vitamin B_6 and vitamin B_{12} have gained particular attention for their cancer-preventive and health-promoting benefits. Highly promising findings about the effects of vitamin D for cancer protection have prompted the American Cancer Society, the American College of Rheumatology, the Canadian Cancer Society, the Canadian Dermatology Association, Dietitians of Canada, the National Council on Skin Cancer Prevention, Osteoporosis Canada and the World Health Organization to recommend daily use of vitamin D supplements or a multivitamin high in vitamin D.

All this being said, you don't necessarily have to take a pile of daily vitamins to reap abundant health rewards, but this chapter should help you to understand the value of my suggested supplements that complete your Hormone Boost plan.

Get the Most Out of Your Supplements

Perhaps I have already convinced you of the importance and health benefits of a few key supplements, and maybe you have gone ahead and purchased a daily vitamin to obtain the nutrients you need for optimal health. Or maybe you've dabbled in supplements for years, and you're now staring at a cupboard full of formulas picked up to deal with everything from belly bloat to aging skin to decreased energy. But how do you know if you're getting the most bang for your buck from your supplements? There are certainly many factors that determine a supplement's quality and absorption. And, unfortunately, not all pills are made equal. There are a few things you ought to consider to improve both the selection and effectiveness of your vitamins:

- **Get alkaline:** Acidity decreases your body's ability to absorb the vitamins and minerals from your food and supplements. It also interferes with your ability to detoxify, disrupts your metabolism and makes you more prone to health problems. To test your levels, purchase pH test strips (available on my website or at any health food store) and test your saliva pH first thing in the morning, one hour before a meal or two hours after eating. Match your strip to the associated color on the package to determine your body pH. Ideally the color on your strip should match the 7.2 to 7.4 range on the package (usually dark green or bluish, depending on the brand of strips you purchase). Remember that processed cereals and flours, sugar, coffee, tea and alcohol are acidifying, whereas vegetables, millet, soy, almonds and wild rice are alkalinizing. By going "greener," you will be improving the absorption of your vitamins and your overall health.
- **Amino acid chelate forms are best for absorption:** Better multivitamins have their vitamins and minerals in highly absorbable forms, like amino acid chelates and citrates, rather than sulfates, carbonates or oxides, although these less absorbable forms are still good for many purposes. Amino acid–bound chelated mineral supplements can provide three to ten times better assimilation than the non-chelated forms. Check labels for the words *glycinate, citrate* or *chelate* to ensure that you are taking the most absorbable

form. Examples include calcium citrate, which is better absorbed than calcium carbonate, and iron glycinate, because it does not cause constipation.

- **Capsules versus tablets:** Capsules are usually more absorbable than tablets because they are easily broken down in the stomach. If tablets are made by a reputable company, however, they are just as absorbable as capsules—and in some cases may be superior. Liquid vitamins and minerals can be the easiest to absorb (especially for children or those who have difficulty swallowing pills), but be sure to avoid the extra sugars or fructose often added to these mixtures to enhance the taste.

- **Avoid fillers:** For best results, look for multivitamins and all other supplement products that are free of binders, fillers, artificial colorings, preservatives, yeast, sugar, starch, hydrogenated oils or other additives. If you suspect food allergies or sensitivities, you may want to be particularly vigilant about looking at your vitamin labels. Lactose, cornstarch, various sugars, soy and yeast can be used as fillers and may cause digestive disturbances in sensitive individuals. In many cases, what you pay for is what you get, so it's worth springing for a product manufactured by a reputable company or purchased through a practitioner's office, as these products are rigorously tested and pure. This is why most people feel and recognize noticeable differences when using products from my Clear Medicine line. They are professional strength and potency, typically are sold only through doctors or pharmacists and are normally much more effective than most health-food store lines.

- **Herbal remedies:** When purchasing an herbal remedy such as valerian or echinacea, ensure that the label says it is "standardized." If a product is standardized, it means it is guaranteed to contain a certain amount of active ingredient. There is a big difference between taking 500 mg of some herb and 500 mg of an herb that is guaranteed to contain 45 percent of the active ingredient. Always be informed about your options and be sure you know what you are looking for.

- **Watch your medications:** A general rule of thumb is that you should take medication at least two hours away from most vitamins, to avoid interactions. A negative interaction may cause a drug-related deficiency of certain nutrients, a loss of potency in medications or a change in the way the drug works in the body. For example, birth control pills typically increase your body's need for B vitamins and folic acid, so you may have to take more of these nutrients to receive the ideal amount. Many antibiotics and chemotherapeutic drugs have interactions with high-dose magnesium and vitamin supplements. Vitamin K (found in liver, broccoli, Brussels sprouts, green leafy vegetables and certain multivitamins) is known to decrease the effects of warfarin, a popular blood thinner. Interactions can also occur between vitamins. For example, you should avoid taking iron with supplements containing calcium, inositol, magnesium, vanadium or vitamin E, since taking them together may interfere with the absorption of one of the supplements. Consult with your pharmacist or doctor when beginning any new medical protocols.

- **Timing is everything:** Remember that the form of the vitamin is important, but the time the vitamin product is taken, in which combinations, and whether or not it is taken with food can also affect a product's effectiveness. A good rule to remember is that vitamins and minerals should generally be taken with food, but herbal supplements are best taken away from food, for optimal absorption and effect. Also, be sure to take your vitamins and minerals away from a fiber supplement, as the combination of the two will decrease overall absorption.

Now that you know what to look for and how to dose yourself, let's move on to some supplements I feel are essential to the Hormone Boost plan, and those that are optional to enhance your results.

The Hormone Boost Supplement Plan

To complement the meal and exercise components of the Hormone Boost plan, a few key supplements will power the six hormones that fuel fat loss and increase strength and energy. I'll give you an overview of these products in this section. You are free to find products with similar ingredients to the Clear Medicine products listed—I include my own formulas because I have witnessed their effectiveness in my practice for over 15 years. Descriptions for each of these products can be found at my online store, which will help if you are looking for comparable products in your area.

Foundation Products

Before we discuss the specific products that will boost the six fat-loss hormones, there are certain foundation products needed to ensure the basics of healthy hormonal balance. Also, they help the Hormone Boost supplements work better. So begin with these:

- **Zinc citrate or polynicotinate, like Clear Zinc 30.** Zinc and magnesium are the most common mineral deficiencies, and zinc helps all of the hormones work better in the body. It has also been proven to assist with weight loss and blood sugar balance. Start with 50 mg per day for 12 weeks (this is the dose recommended in the study that found zinc helped weight loss), then reduce the dosage to 25 mg or less, perhaps by taking a lower-dose zinc supplement or a multivitamin, or by using a meal replacement daily, such as Clear Complete, that has a multivitamin with zinc in the formula.
- **Magnesium glycinate (capsule), like Clear Magnesium Calm.** Most adults are deficient in magnesium, a mineral essential for healthy sleep, digestive support, blood sugar

and insulin balance and metabolism. Because magnesium is involved in over 300 enzymatic reactions in the body, failing to have enough means your metabolic processes slow down on a cellular level. Eventually this manifests on a physical level as metabolism slows and energy plummets. Take 200 to 600 mg at bedtime (this is one to five capsules of my formula) or use a topical magnesium chloride spray and apply four sprays on each limb.

- **Omega supplement, like Clear Omega (marine-sourced omegas) or Pure Form Omega (plant-based omegas).** This supplement helps your brain and virtually every single cell in your body, because all cell membranes are made up of the phospholipids from fats. The healthier your fat intake, the healthier your cell membranes (and hormone receptors) will be. Take four capsules per day of Clear Omega (extra-strength EPA/DHA from fish oil) or Pure Form Omega (my favorite plant-based omega). I guarantee you will never experience oil "repeat" after swallowing either of these products.
- **A high-potency probiotic for healthy digestion and immune support, like Clear Flora.** Remember that your gut is closely involved in the ability to lose fat, balance blood sugar, activate hormones, reduce inflammation and eliminate harmful hormonal waste. Take one capsule upon rising of Clear Flora refrigerated formula (sold as a glass bottle of capsules, each providing 15 billion live bacterial) or Clear Flora non-refrigerated (sold in a box containing 30 capsules, each providing 30 billion live bacterial), which is great for travel and for promoting bowel regularity.
- **Basic antioxidants, like Clear C Boost and Clear E Boost.** You can consume these by sourcing each from individual supplements, in an antioxidant combo product, in a multivitamin or in a meal replacement that includes vitamins. My vitamin C contains 7.5 mg of black pepper extract, called bioperine

(which increases its bioavailability) along with 750 mg of vitamin C (not sourced from corn, like many products on the market). Clear E Boost contains all eight types of vitamin E, including a potent dose of gamma E that offers benefits for breast cancer protection.

If you want to make smoothies or protein meal replacements part of your plan, you may also need:

- **Protein supplement:** Choose from whey, rice, pea, hemp or another vegan protein option. You need protein to boost the fat-burning, muscle-building and appetite-controlling hormones. You also need protein to support liver detoxification, immune function and the growth and maintenance of muscle tissue—as well as for healthy skin, hair and nails.
- **Dream Protein:** A long-time favorite whey protein brand at my clinic and my online store for years, Dream Protein is cold-filtered and free of artificial sweeteners and glutamate (a neurotoxic compound in some protein supplements). Use 1.5 to 2 scoops per smoothie.
- **Clear Complete:** A complete meal replacement to use as an on-the-go option, Clear Complete contains protein, carb, fat and fiber as well as a multivitamin (including the zinc, magnesium and vitamins C and E listed earlier). You can also use this product to make your Hormone Boost plan as simple as possible; use 1.5 to 2 scoops of Clear Complete for two meals per day and consume solid foods for the other two meals. As a vegan alternative, look for my Clear Vegan – Protein Complete Cleanse (use 1–1.5 scoops.)
- **Clear Fiber:** I recommend using fiber supplements in smoothies to provide the highest amount of fiber needed to stimulate an adiponectin boost and support healthy digestion. I love Clear Fiber—it is a mixture of non-irritating

soluble and insoluble fiber to assist with bowel regularity. Add 1 to 2 scoops to your smoothies daily.

- **Hemp seeds or olive oil:** These are my preferred fat sources for smoothies. Hemp seeds contain GLA and additional protein to boost fat loss, and olive oil has been proven to be more beneficial for fat loss when consumed at breakfast. So have olive oil in your shake at breakfast and hemp seeds in your shake if you have another at your 3 to 4 p.m. meal. (Check out my smoothie kit at my online store, and on-the-go protein kit options too.)

- **B-UP Bars:** "Over the years, the biggest criticism of protein bars has been the inclusion of so many hard-to-pronounce ingredients that sound like they are straight from an AP chemistry class. Who knows the effect they have on your physique, much less your colon? The new gluten-free B-UP protein bar is a lean, mean, protein-delivering machine that contains only 12 ingredients. Its 20 g of protein are derived from whey and milk protein isolate, a very pure form of protein that has been stripped of almost all of its carbs, fats and lactose. Studies have also shown that whey protein isolate blunts hunger hormones and promotes satiety, making it one of the **smartest protein choices** when you're cutting calories. Each bar is loaded with prebiotic fiber and delivers just 4 g of impact carbs. If you're on a diet, this bar is your new best friend." This is an excerpt from *Iron Man* magazine, which rated B-UP as the best protein bar of 2016. I am very picky when it comes to bars—and this one fits the Hormone Boost nutritional guidelines.

If you want to include the Hormone Boost fasting day in your plan—and I highly recommend that you do—you will need:

- **Clear Cleanse – intermittent fasting support**. Have one scoop in one quart of water, four times a day. Alternatively, you can use herbal teas—a mix of ginger, lemon, green tea, etc.—to make your own cleanse-day formula.

The first five supplements listed in this section are the absolute musts; the next five I list could be essentials, depending on how you want to shape your plan.

Boost Products

Now that we've covered the foundation products, we're ready to move on to the supplements that are my favorite choices to power up your fat-loss hormones. You can select the supplement to match the hormones you want to boost, or you can boost all of them if you wish. If your supplement budget allows, incorporating these will accelerate your results. Again, there is no pressure to buy the Clear Medicine formulations; alternative products are absolutely viable as long as they contain similar ingredients (and I recommend doing a bit of research on the brand itself to ensure organic ingredients and practices).

- **Clear Detox – Hormonal Health:** Use this to support liver function, get rid of toxins and hormonal waste (especially harmful estrogen) and combat inflammation. Healthy liver function is especially important because it activates thyroid and growth hormones. Take one dose at breakfast, or at lunch if you are taking a thyroid medication upon rising. If you cannot afford all the supplements in this section, this is the one to buy.
- **Clear Energy – Dopamine Support Formula:** Use this for a thyroid, dopamine and adrenaline boost. Take three capsules upon rising.
- **Clear Balance – Stress Support Formula:** Use this for a DHEA and testosterone boost and stress support. Take one capsule upon rising and two before bed.
- **Clear ZZZ's – Melatonin:** Use this to boost melatonin, thyroid

hormone and growth hormone. Take 1.5 to 3 lozenges a half-hour before bedtime.

- **Clear Recovery – Sports and Energy Formula:** This will boost growth hormone. Take half a scoop in water before or after a workout or before bed.

Did you notice that specific supplements for adiponectin and glucagon are not listed here? That's because you can obtain a fantastic increase in these via the Hormone Boost nutrition plan (glucagon from increased protein in your diet; adiponectin from increased fiber). Should you wish to give yourself an additional boost, you are free to consider the supplement options I have included in Chapters 5 and 6.

Visit my website to download a daily vitamin dosing sheet that you can stick on your fridge, with easy references to keep you on track.

You've got your food and fuel lined up; so now let's take things to the next level with your Hormone Boost workout.

A HORMONE BOOST REAL-LIFE SUCCESS STORY

THE CLIENT: Michelle C.

DETAILS: Female, 49

BODY COMPOSITION RESULTS (FROM SCALE AND BODY FAT/MUSCLE MASS VIA BIO-IMPEDANCE TESTING)

MEASUREMENT	BEFORE	AFTER	TOTAL LOSS/GAIN
Weight (lb.)	145	133	(-) 12
Lean Body Mass (lb.)	101.8	102.8	(+) 1
Fat Mass (lb.)	43.2	31	(-) 12.2
Basal Metabolic Rate (calories/day)	1,441 calories	1,465 calories	(+) 24

Michelle, another of the women I treated on the *Marilyn Denis Show*, was a perfect example of the craving, bloated and belly-fat type; she was taking the birth-control pill and had tons of cravings, water retention and abdominal bloating. After six weeks on the Hormone Boost plan, she lost 12 pounds of fat and gained one pound of muscle! (You can watch the show here: www.marilyn.ca/mobile/Segment?segid=109608.)

CHAPTER 12

THE HORMONE BOOST WORKOUT

*Twenty years from now, you will be more disappointed by
the things that you didn't do than by the ones you did do, so throw
off the bowlines, sail away from safe harbor, catch the trade winds
in your sails. Explore. Dream. Discover.*

MARK TWAIN

There is conflicting evidence on how our hormones affect the results of our workouts. There is no doubt, however, that how we exercise and the activities we choose absolutely impact our hormones. When done correctly and often enough, exercise boosts almost all six of the fat-loss hormones—and the mood hormones too. It is definitely a vital component of the Hormone Boost plan, whether you decide to start right away or a few weeks into your Boost.

The effects of exercise on your hormones and your weight will vary depending on the type of activities you choose (cardio, weight training or yoga) and the intensity and duration of your sessions. But no matter what type of exercise you do, working out is just plain good for you. Here's why:

- **It burns calories:** We burn calories while we exercise and, if we do strength training, we burn calories well after the session is completed too. High-intensity strength training can actually help you burn extra calories for *up to 72 hours* after your workout.

- **It builds muscle:** Exercise can help us build metabolically active muscle. For every pound of muscle you gain, you'll burn extra calories, even when you're doing absolutely nothing!

- **It stimulates muscle-building hormones:** A study published in the *Journals of Gerontology, Series A: Biological Sciences and Medical Sciences* (2002) looked at hormonal changes occurring in menopausal women who completed endurance training (40 minutes of cycling at 75 percent maximal exertion) and resistance training (3 sets of 10 reps of 8 exercises), compared with a control group that didn't exercise. Both endurance and resistance training increased estrogen, testosterone and growth hormone significantly. Only the resistance training, however, increased DHEA. Testosterone levels will rise higher when you play a competitive sport, and even higher still if you win.

- **It reduces our fat-loss foes:** Exercise reduces the hormones that interfere with fat loss, including excess stress hormones (which can wear the body down) and excess estrogen (which can increase breast cancer risk). Researchers selected a group of postmenopausal women from Seattle who did not exercise. Half were instructed to begin a moderate-intensity walking program (45 minutes five times a week); half were told to do only stretching exercises. The women walking *decreased* their harmful estrogen within three months.

- **It's a mood booster:** Exercise stimulates your mood and mental function, decreases anxiety and depression and reduces pain by increasing dopamine and endorphins, our natural painkillers. According to a 2005 study from the *European Journal of Sports Science,* just 15 minutes of cardiovascular exercise two to three times a week can boost serotonin enough to prevent anxiety and treat depression.

- **It burns fat and balances insulin:** Exercise cranks up our PPARs (peroxisome proliferator-activated receptors), the regulators of fat metabolism and insulin sensitivity in our muscle cells.
- **It controls appetite and reduces inflammation:** Exercise has positive effects on the fat-cell hormones, such as leptin and adiponectin, that control inflammation and influence our appetite.

Exercise is the key for your head, just as it is for your heart. It has a unique capacity to exhilarate and relax, to provide stimulation and calm, to counter depression and dissipate stress. I believe exercise is the number one way to change your life. Its restorative powers and mood-enhancing effects have been verified in clinical trials that have used exercise to treat anxiety and depression. The mental benefits of exercise actually have a hormonal basis—it reduces stress hormones and stimulates the production of endorphins, the body's natural painkillers and mood elevators.

Meanwhile, the act of exercising (that is, the behaviors related to it) contribute to the emotional benefits. As your waistline shrinks and your strength and stamina increase, your self-image will improve. You'll earn a sense of pride and self-confidence. Your renewed vigor will help you succeed in many tasks, and the discipline you practice on this front will help you achieve other lifestyle goals. Exercise and sports also provide opportunities to either enjoy some solitude or make friends and build networks. Sounds good? I think so—and I've devised a schedule to help you do it.

The Hormone Boost Workout Weekly Schedule

For maximum health and hormonal benefits, I recommend that you exercise six days a week. You'll complete three types of workouts each week (and you'll see the rationale for each of these activities in the coming pages): (1) yoga, (2) walking and/or interval cardio and (3) strength training.

I believe it's important to schedule your workouts—including your walks—because it really helps you stick with them. The workout program here is designed to keep you working hard during each session and progressing each week, allowing specific muscle groups to recuperate while others are being pushed to develop. Before we get into specifics, though, let's look at each type of workout and the benefits it provides.

The Yoga Boost

With its full spectrum of poses, yoga can bring the body back into its natural alignment, level out muscular imbalances and improve physical weaknesses. If you are an athlete, yoga can improve your performance by enhancing your flexibility, relaxation, breathing and balance. And anyone can improve posture, energy and endurance with regular yoga practice. Yoga offers fabulous benefits for calming your nervous system, restoring hormonal balance *and* strengthening your muscles.

Yoga is also a terrific stress reliever. Numerous studies, including one completed in 2003 by the Myrna Brind Center for Integrative Medicine (at Thomas Jefferson University) and the Yoga Research Society, have shown that yoga can lower blood cortisol levels in healthy men and women. It is also known to reduce adrenaline and stimulate the calming brain chemical GABA. Research from Boston University School of Medicine and McLean Hospital (*Journal of Alternative and Complementary Medicine*, May 2007) suggests yoga should be explored as a possible treatment for disorders often associated with low GABA levels, such as depression and anxiety.

Yoga's benefits extend even further; a study conducted by Ohio State University and published in *Psychosomatic Medicine* (January 2010) indicates that yoga may even act to reduce inflammation in the body. In this research, 50 subjects were divided into two groups: a group of regular yoga practitioners and a group of beginners.

Researchers assessed blood samples from each of the subjects and found that those in the novice group had 41 percent higher levels of an inflammatory compound called interleukin-6, compared to their more advanced peers.

If you struggle with excess belly fat or sleep disruption, yoga is a stellar workout choice. It's also excellent if you have fertility concerns. For all these reasons, it is included in your Hormone Boost plan. A yoga class or a yoga DVD at home are both excellent options. As far as the type of yoga is concerned, I prefer hatha or ashtanga, but whatever form works best for you and your body is the one you should choose. Note, though, that it is best to avoid yoga (especially power yoga) on the same day as you do weights, since it can cause too much muscle strain.

Walking for a Boost

Even a short stroll can be a simple and highly beneficial way to avoid falling off the track with your diet—and lessen the harmful effects of stress and fatty foods on your body. Walking after an unhealthy meal can curb the effects of stress by reducing the amounts of fatty acids, sugars and stress hormones that are released into the bloodstream and subsequently stored as fat. This gentle form of exercise strengthens nearly every aspect of your body, promotes energy during the day, encourages a relaxation response and improves the quality of your sleep.

Another plus: Walking boosts adiponectin when we do it a minimum of three times per week. According to a study published in the *American Diabetes Journal* (2010), adiponectin levels rose by 260 percent after two to three bouts of exercise per week *and* remained elevated after 10 weeks. The data indicate that elevated adiponectin levels are first apparent after one week (two to three bouts) of moderately intense exercise. Isn't it amazing how quickly the body responds when we give it the right stimuli?

Strength Training: A Hormone Boost Must!

I have been preaching the benefits of strength training since I fixed my metabolism and polycystic ovarian syndrome with it in 1999. The effect this kind of exercise has on our hormones is truly remarkable. Case in point: Researchers found that strength training improved muscle quality and whole-body insulin sensitivity. Decreased inflammation and increased adiponectin levels were also associated with improved metabolic control. By now you're aware that high adiponectin blood levels are linked with a reduced risk of heart attack, while low levels are often found in people who are obese—and at *increased* risk of heart attack.

The metabolic equation is very simple; the more muscle tissue you have, the better your metabolism and the more calories you will burn. Even the process of breaking down and repairing your muscles post-workout increases your metabolism. Dr. Miriam Nelson, a Tufts University researcher, showed that a group of women who followed a weight-loss diet and did weight-training exercises lost 44 percent more fat than those who only followed the diet.

While aerobic activity can help burn calories during the activity, building muscle via strength training means you will *continue* to burn more calories, even while you sleep. And doing your cardio sessions right after your strength training will render even better results. A study from the College of New Jersey confirms that pumping iron or even lifting your own body weight can make your cardio workout more effective. Participants who performed an intense weight workout before riding a stationary bike burned more fat during their cardio session than those who pedaled but skipped the weights. So remember to do your cardio sessions either immediately after your weight training or on a separate day, never before and not for too long.

It has long been established that the *right* exercise increases your ability to transport sugar into the tissues rather than let it build up in the blood. This effect can be seen even in previously sedentary adults. In fact, according to an article published in the *New England Journal of Medicine* (1996), a single session of moderate-intensity exercise can improve blood sugar balance by at least 40 percent. This impact isn't permanent, however, since the effects of exercise diminish within 48 to 72 hours. *This research supports my recommendation of a program that includes strength training three days a week and walking three to five times a week.* This regimen will have a profound impact on your levels of all six fat-burning hormone—not to mention your body composition.

The type of weight training in the Hormone Boost exercise plan stems from German Body Composition Training (GBCT). After working with my friend and trainer Mike Demeter, I quickly discovered how effective these workouts are for building muscle and dropping fat—often a tough combo to achieve. This type of training was popularized by Charles Poliquin in his book *German Body Comp Program: Burn Fat and Build Muscle on the Only Program That Uses Weight Training for Weight Loss* (2004), and it originates from research by a Romanian exercise scientist named Hala Rambie.

Rambie made the important discovery that the lactic acid metabolic pathway is better for fat loss than the commonly accepted aerobic pathway. He found that high blood lactic levels decrease blood pH levels, which in turn sends a message to the brain to accelerate its production of growth hormone. And you and I both know that higher growth hormone counts increase fat loss (if you need a refresher on this, see Chapter 4). We have confirmed that growth hormone is linked to lactate production by looking at studies involving patients with a metabolic disorder that makes them unable to produce lactate during exercise. Without the lactic acid boost, no changes in growth hormone status were observed in study participants (*British Journal of Sports Medicine*, July 2009).

To achieve these fat-loss and hormone-enhancing results, GBCT—and Hormone Boost—workouts use short rest intervals and multi-joint (often full-body) movements to generate maximum growth hormone production. This not only results in greater fat loss than aerobic programs can produce, but (more importantly) it also will not sacrifice strength and muscle mass. For creation of the actual workouts, I had the pleasure of calling on one of my Clear Medicine team members—Anthony Boudreau. He is our resident strength-training expert, and our clients have loved him for years!

A BOOST IN BONE HEALTH

One summer at my family cottage in Nova Scotia, my grandmother, Mrs. Mary Rivers, was hugged by a long-time friend who popped in (by the way, everyone does the "drop-in" down there, something I sometimes miss, living in Toronto). Poor Nan! The pressure from the gentleman's embrace broke her rib. A few years later, she suffered a spontaneous fracture in her spine, an injury that kept her mostly confined to a horizontal position and unable to go up stairs for the last nine years of her life. Incredibly, I never once heard her complain.

My family's experience with osteoporosis—or bone-density loss—didn't end with her. Both my mom and Uncle Bruce, her brother, have it now, and I have had evidence of bone-density loss on scans in the past (before I implemented proper strength training). Although my intention was to avoid including negative health stats or study findings in this book, this topic is too important to ignore. More women die each year as a result of osteoporotic fractures than from breast and ovarian cancer combined. I saw this statistic and, with my personal experience, knew I needed to add a bone boost to the Hormone Boost plan. These are some of the surprising facts about osteoporosis:

- *Osteoporosis* and *osteopenia* (bone loss before the development of full-blown osteoporosis) affect over 3.2 million people in Canada (more than 10 percent of the population).

- According to the International Osteoporosis Foundation, osteo-porosis and low bone mass are currently estimated to be a major public health threat for almost 44 million American women and men aged 50 and older, which equates to 55 percent of that population segment in the United States. About 54 percent of postmenopausal white women in the United States have osteo-penia, and 30 percent have osteoporosis.
- According to Osteoporosis Canada, the overall yearly cost to the Canadian health-care system of treating osteoporosis and its associated fractures was over $2.3 billion as of 2010. This includes acute-care costs, outpatient care, prescription drugs and indirect costs. This amount rises to $3.9 billion if a proportion of Canadians are assumed to be living in long-term care facilities because of osteoporosis (*Osteoporosis International*, March 2012). Caring for these fractures in the United States and Europe is just as expensive; the International Osteoporosis Foundation (www.capturethefracture.org) reports a cost of US $20 billion and €32 billion, respectively.

Although we don't often think of it this way, bone is living tissue. It's composed of hydroxylapatite crystals, made of calcium and phosphorus, which are deposited on collagen fibers. Other minerals are also deposited to form a matrix. This structure, much like steel-reinforced concrete, gives bone its incredible strength and resilience. Bone is, therefore, *a constant work in progress*, built up by the cells that make bones (osteoblasts) and torn down by cells that break down bones (osteoclasts). As we age, the process of rebuilding bone slows down, which means that we lose bone and it becomes porous. As bone becomes weak, even a small trauma can result in debilitat-ing fractures. Because peak bone mass is reached during young adulthood, and we know that improved bone mass reduces the risk of osteoporosis, optimal bone-building nutrition is essential from childhood into your 30s (*Journal of Nutrition*, 1996).

When it comes to dealing with osteoporosis, I am not sure which is worse—the disease itself or the conventional treatment of it. Medications currently on the market to improve this condition are wrought with the severe risk of side effects and even the risk of complete treatment failure. For instance, the bisphosphonate drugs, including Fosamax, prescribed for osteoporosis are proven to increase the risk of femur fracture and cause bone formation that is not, in fact, healthy bone. These drugs are also known to produce serious gastrointestinal side effects, so troublesome that up to 30 percent of people cannot take them.

Obviously, osteoporosis is a weakening condition that needs chronic, long-term and focused efforts for its prevention and subsequent treatment. In my mind, this means a multifaceted approach (which is what I recommend for all chronic conditions). Taking a single approach for the management of age-related diseases is impractical; improving bone health is no different. Case in point: While many of us are fully aware of the importance of taking calcium and magnesium to reduce the risk of osteoporosis, those two nutrients are by no means enough. If you are concerned about preserving bone health or currently have osteoporosis, bone up on the following tips to use along with the rest of the Hormone Boost plan.

Nutrition Tips for Bone Health

- **Eat Mediterranean:** The incidence of osteoporosis is lower in Mediterranean areas than other European countries. The explanation may lie partly in the traditional Mediterranean diet, which is rich in fruits, vegetables and olive oil. One study in the Endocrine Society's *Journal of Clinical Endocrinology & Metabolism* (October 2012) revealed that consumption of a Mediterranean diet enriched with olive oil (compared to a low-fat diet) for two years is associated with increased serum osteocalcin concentrations, suggesting a protective effect on bone. All the more reason to include a tablespoon of olive oil in your meals, twice daily.

- **Get your greens and reds:** Research from the *American Journal of Clinical Nutrition* (September 2005) suggests that 10 servings of fruits and vegetables per day help to build bone density, offering yet another reason to get your recommended daily servings. If you have children, help them form this habit too. Researchers at the University of Saskatchewan found that boys who ate the most fruits and vegetables showed the greatest accumulation of mineral in their bones throughout childhood and adolescence, which translates to denser, stronger bones. Boys who consumed 10 servings of fruits and vegetables a day wound up accumulating 48.6 g more mineral content in their bones than boys who ate just a single serving. Fruits and vegetables are rich in the minerals required to control acid levels in the body, and thus prevent bone loss, as well as plant-sourced vitamin K, which is involved in bone cell formation. Do you struggle to get your daily dose? Go for Clear Greens in the water that you take your probiotic with daily. It can help with regulating your body pH balance too.

Lifestyle Tips for Bone Health

- **The Hormone Boost strength-training workout—JUST DO IT!** Bone density has a lot to do with what you do—or do not do—at the gym. Bone tissue is always changing because to hormonal fluctuations and physical activity (or lack thereof). Regular strength training helps to deposit more minerals in the bones, especially those in the legs, hips and spine. The opposite is also true; lack of regular exercise will accelerate bone loss. One study in the Endocrine Society's *Journal of Clinical Endocrinology & Metabolism* (2012) suggests that physical activity for premenopausal women is very effective in reducing sclerostin, a known inhibitor of bone formation. The study found that women who had *more than two hours of physical activity per week* had significantly lower levels of serum sclerostin, and higher IGF-1 levels (your youthful hormone), than women who had less than two hours of physical activity per week.

- **Balance your sex and strength hormones:** The decline in your sex hormones—estrogen, progesterone and testosterone—with age accelerates bone loss. Here's why: As we've seen, the two important cell types in bone tissue, osteoblasts and osteoclasts, work to produce new bone tissue and remove existing bone tissue, respectively. Without enough estrogen, osteoclast activity speeds up and bones lose their density. Progesterone and testosterone have been shown to stimulate osteoblast activity and potentially aid new bone growth. Revisit my suggestions in Chapter 9 (Step Three: Give Your Sex Life a Boost).

- **Go natural to boost serotonin:** One major downside of antidepressants is their link to osteoporosis. Two new studies suggest that older men and women taking SSRIs—a class of antidepressants that includes Prozac, Paxil and Zoloft—are prone to increased bone loss, according to Oregon Health & Science University findings (June 2007). While people experiencing clinical depression should never go off meds without medical supervision, I recommend that the rest of us look for natural ways to manage a serotonin boost. Plenty of sunlight, a healthy diet rich in protein, minerals and vitamins, regular exercise and good sleep support serotonin production. You can also use natural alternatives like high-dose fish oil (Clear Omega, twice daily), vitamin D (Clear D_3 drops) (4,000 to 5,000 IU daily) and 5-HTP (Clear Mood, 2 at bedtime and 1 at breakfast). More news on serotonin can be found in Chapter 7.

- **Tighten your belt buckle**: If you are prone to osteoporosis, you may be shocked to discover that all the calcium in the world isn't going to help you maintain your bones—if your insulin levels are high. In fact, most of that calcium will be eliminated through your urine or, even worse, form calcifications in your arteries. In an important feedback loop, insulin signals osteoblasts to activate a hormone called osteocalcin, which in turn promotes glucose metabolism. Coupled with weight gain caused by insulin resistance, calcium loss and surging insulin both increase your chances of breaking or fracturing a bone. This is just one reason why the Hormone Boost diet is essential—it keeps your insulin levels low!

- **B is for bone health**: Homocysteine is an inflammatory protein that, if elevated in the blood, is a proven independent risk factor for osteoporosis as well as heart disease, Alzheimer's and strokes. Homocysteine has also been found to increase with insulin resistance and is a sign of B vitamin deficiency, according to the results of a study in the June 2008 issue of the *Journal of Clinical Endocrinology & Metabolism*. Get your vitamin B levels (B_{12}, B_6 and folic acid) and homocysteine tested, and if your homocysteine is above 6.3, I recommend including a complex of vitamin B_6, vitamin B_{12} and folic acid (such as B_{12} lozenges from Biotics Research or Clear B boost) in your daily vitamin regimen for at least three months, or until your next physical exam, when you should repeat the blood test.

Supplement Tips for Bone Health

- The Hormone Boost foundation supplements (see Chapter 11) all contribute to bone health generally, but I'll outline their benefits specifically.
  - > Vitamin D_3: Adequate vitamin D and calcium intake is the cornerstone of osteoporosis prevention and treatment. Vitamin D intake between 500 and 800 IU daily, with or without calcium supplementation, has been shown to increase bone mineral density in women with a mean age of approximately 63 years, though I normally recommend 2,000 to 5,000 IU daily. I suggest not taking vitamin D alone, however, since there's insufficient data to support a benefit from vitamin D supplementation without calcium to prevent osteoporotic fracture in postmenopausal women (*Journal of Women's Health*, March 2003).

> Select a plant-based omega like Pure Form Omega as your omega source. According to a study in the *Journal of Nutrition* (June 2011), protective associations were observed between intakes of alpha-linolenic acid (ALA) and hip fracture risk in a combined sample of women and men. Participants with the highest ALA intake had a 54 percent lower risk of hip fracture. Take two capsules twice daily.

> Look for a multi-mineral supplement that contains all the essentials for bone health, including boron and vitamin K_2 (e.g., Ortho Bone or Ortho Minerals from AOR), and take three capsules twice daily. Add more magnesium glycinate at bedtime; it helps bone density, metabolism and sleep.

> Antioxidant vitamins E and C manage inflammation and collagen, which is important for bone health. Vitamin C also protects the immune system and helps your body handle stress.

- A lozenge of B_{12}, B_6 and folic acid will provide the B vitamins needed for bone health and homocysteine metabolism. My favorite is the B_{12} lozenge from Biotics Research. It is so absorbable that many of my patients only need one every other day, but it can be used daily. Suck it; don't chew!

- Include conjugated linoleic acid (CLA) in your vitamin regimen. CLA has been shown to help preserve lean muscle as well as maintain bone density and muscle mass and improve insulin balance (*Journal of the American College of Nutrition*, June 2005). Take two capsules twice daily.

- Melatonin: I have outlined the benefits of melatonin for bone health in Chapter 7. Take a 3 mg lozenge at bedtime.

- Clear Recovery: Use this for a supply of the amino acids that aid growth hormone overnight. Have 1/2 scoop in water at bedtime. You can add it to the same fluid you use to swallow your minerals.

- Balance DHEA and cortisol with Clear Balance – Stress Support Formula. Clear Balance contains Relora, which has been shown in studies to increase DHEA and reduce cortisol (which tears down bone) in just two to four weeks of use. You may recall the benefits of DHEA and testosterone for bone health from an earlier discussion in Chapter 3. Take two Clear Balance capsules at bedtime and one upon rising.

The Hormone Boost Exercise Guidelines

Before you begin, let's go through the general rules of the Hormone Boost exercise plan. Those of you who have been following me since *The Hormone Diet* will recognize them—they are the same! It's been almost 10 years since I first shared that workout, and it's still the perfect way to achieve optimal results.

- **Keep it short and sweet.** All workouts are 30 minutes (maximum 40 minutes).
- **Give every workout your all.** High intensity and maximum effort—to the point where you just can't squeeze out one more rep—is a *must* for effective fat-burning and hormonal benefits. You can push yourself this hard in the gym (or wherever you exercise) because you know your workout is short and it will soon be over!
- **Complete your exercises with a short rest between each circuit.** Circuit training keeps your heart rate high throughout your workout. When you use this method, you basically get your cardio workout and strength training all in one shorter session. Circuit training is also the best type of workout for improving insulin response, boosting testosterone and stimulating growth hormone. So you spend less time exercising but you reap even more benefits.
- **Work multiple muscle groups with each strength-training session (each muscle group should be trained only once or twice a week).** This approach is designed to increase growth

hormone and stimulate more muscle groups at once. It also lets you complete more work in less time and ensures that your muscles get the proper recuperation time they need between sessions.

- **Walking or interval cardio is best for the Hormone Boost (bike rides, rollerblading, etc., are done for fun).** Intervals are short periods of intense exercise separated by periods of brief rest or lighter activity. This method of training offers the most fat-burning potential and the greatest health benefits. It increases the intensity of your training too, which once again means greater benefits from less time spent exercising. Even cardiac patients can use interval training to improve their fitness. Walking provides the greatest boost of adiponectin when we do it rigorously at least three times per week.
- **Use yoga for its hormone-boosting effects.** Besides challenging and stretching your muscles, yoga can improve blood sugar metabolism and insulin balance and stimulate brain-calming GABA.
- **Consume the right stuff before and after your workouts.** Always consume a blend of protein and carbohydrate about one hour before and within 45 minutes after your resistance-training sessions. Limit fat in your post-workout meal. This combination is proven to stimulate more growth hormone release and encourage muscle gains. You can do cardio on an empty stomach (though you don't have to), but eat your snack of protein and carbs (again, no fat) within 45 minutes of finishing your session. Drink only water during your workouts—no sports drinks allowed!

Tools of the Trade

Whether you choose to work out in the gym, outside or at home, you'll need a few key pieces of equipment to get the job done properly. Most gyms provide these items for you, but you can also purchase them yourself for more flexible workouts.

- **A set of dumbbells:** 3, 5, 8, 10, 12 and 15 pounds for women; 10, 15, 20, 25 and 30 pounds for men.
- **A support bench:** A weight bench or other stable bench is helpful, but not necessary if you have a stability ball.
- **Options for indoor cardio:** A stationary bike, treadmill, stepper or elliptical machine for home use. (You can also walk, bike or run outside when weather permits.)
- **Music:** Listening to your favorite tunes while working out can be a great motivator—and offer real hormonal benefits too!

Selecting the Right Amount of Weight

Time and time again I see people at the gym who fail to get results, either because they don't lift enough weight to challenge their muscles or because they're lifting too much and using improper form. Choosing the right weight and using the correct form are absolutely *essential* to get the results you want and avoid injury.

When you are just starting out, choose a weight light enough to allow you to complete all the suggested repetitions for each exercise *without compromising your form*. Remember, if your posture is poor or you are swinging your weights instead of lifting

Exercise is proven to combat the loss of muscle that unfortunately but inevitably happens with aging. But here's some good news: According to research from the Public Library of Science (plos.org), supplements of creatine monohydrate (5 g per day) and conjugated linoleic acid (CLA; 3 to 6 g per day) can boost the benefits of exercise even further. Naturally produced by our body and present in meat, creatine is known to supply our muscles with energy. CLA, a naturally occurring fatty acid in beef, helps to preserve muscle tissue while encouraging safe fat loss. When used in conjunction with exercise, these two supplements pack a powerful muscle-building and anti-aging punch.

Get Fit Quick with CLA and Creatine

them in a controlled manner, just to finish the last few reps, you're not doing yourself any favors! In fact, you can really hurt yourself—not to mention that you're not getting the workout you intended. As your workouts progress, you'll decrease the number of repetitions and increase your weight to the point where you can barely complete the last few repetitions.

Hiring a personal trainer may seem like a daunting or expensive proposition, but don't be afraid to try it, even for just a few sessions, if you feel you need help getting started or guidance on proper form. (Note: Some trainers will charge less if you do your session with a partner, so find a workout buddy!) We're talking about an investment in your long-term health and well-being. I fully believe it's some of the best money you will ever spend and I encourage all my patients to do so.

The Plan

Now that you know you simply *have* to exercise for lasting metabolic and hormonal health, let's lay out the exact workout plan to help you do it.

MONDAY	TUESDAY	WEDNESDAY	THURSDAY
Rest	Strength-Training Session, Day 1	Cardio Interval Training * Yoga	Strength-Training Session, Day 2

FRIDAY	SATURDAY	SUNDAY	
Yoga	Strength-Training Session, Day 3	Cardio (Optional: 20–40 minutes of cardio at a steady pace or interval)*	

* Walk three to five times per week, complete interval training one to two times per week, or choose a mix of both depending on the timing and energy level of your day.

- Do yoga once or twice a week.
- The three weekly strength-training workouts are outlined on pages 239 to 241. Instructions for the movements are available online at www.drnatashaturner.com, in the "Book Extras" section for *The Hormone Boost*.
- Although not specifically scheduled, walking should be part of your routine a minimum of four days a week, for 40 to 60 minutes at a time. There is no maximum for walking— you can do it daily if you wish. I like to wear 2.5-pound wrist and ankle weights, and I prefer to walk outside. If you walk on a treadmill, do not hold on and make sure you up the incline to a minimum of level one. If you do not want to walk or are short on time, include one or two sprinting or interval-training sessions per week.

The Hormone Boost Strength-Training Workout

As we learned earlier, the goal of the GBCT program is to produce as much lactic acid as possible. The more lactic acid you produce, the more growth hormone you produce, and with that increase in growth hormone comes greater fat loss—the exact results the Hormone Boost is striving for. The quickest way to start this cascade of events is to use multi-joint exercises with short rest intervals. If done properly, your heart rate will climb, your muscles will burn and you will sweat.

Before we get into the specifics of the program designed by my strength and conditioning expert, Anthony Boudreau, it's imperative to understand the following guidelines:

- Choose a weight that will cause you to "max out" by the time you approach the end of the set (i.e., you just can't do another rep). If your muscles aren't burning and shaking, then increase the weight—but make sure you perform the exercises with proper form and technique.

- Be sure to respect the rest period so that you can reach maximal effort and results from your workouts; 30 seconds is just enough time to switch exercises, and 60 seconds is enough time to allow you to recover before you start the circuit over again.
- You should perform each session outlined here once a week, but if done properly with the Hormone Boost nutrition, supplement and recovery guidelines, four times per week just might be your secret advantage in becoming the better you—*fast*.

Finally, here is some explanation of Anthony's workout terms for your complete understanding:

- **Exercise Order:** The letter and number combo you'll see in the strength-training charts refers to exercise groups. You must complete all sets of A exercises before moving on to the B exercises. If there is a number with a number and letter, alternate between these exercises during the workout (e.g., A1 and A2). So you will complete a set of A1, a set of A2 and then a set of A1 and A2 again, and again—for a total of 3 sets each.
- **Tempo:** The tempo is a four-number sequence that dictates the speed at which you will perform each part of the movement. More specifically:
  - > The first number is the eccentric movement—when you lower the weight.
  - > The second number is the point where you need to pause to change the direction, from lowering to lifting the weight.
  - > The third number is the concentric movement—when you lift the weight.
  - > The fourth number is the point where you change the direction, from lifting to lowering the weight.

So, for example, 3-1-2-0 means: down for 3, pause 1, up in 2, no pause, repeat.

- **Sets:** This is the number of cycles of reps that you will do.
- **Reps:** This is the number of times you will do one complete motion of an exercise.
- **Rest:** This is the time you have to rest, in seconds, between exercises.
- **Weight:** You can fill in the weights you are lifting and change them, if needed, as you progress.

STRENGTH-TRAINING SESSION, DAY 1					
EXERCISE	TEMPO	SETS	REPS	REST	WEIGHT (LBS)
A1) Deadlift	4-1-1-0/ 4-0-1-0	3	10–12	30 seconds	
A2) Push-ups/Dips	3-0-1-0	3	10–12/ 8–10	60 seconds	
B1) Bridge/Hip Thrust	3-0-1-1	3	10–12	30 seconds	
B2) Standing Shoulder Press/ Push Press	3-0-1-0	3	10–12	60 seconds	
C1) Hamstring Curl/ Glute Ham Developer	4-0-1-0/ 3-0-1-0	3	8–10	30 seconds	
C2) Incline Dumbbell Press/ Landmine Press	3-0-1-0	3	10–12	60 seconds	

STRENGTH-TRAINING SESSION, DAY 2					
EXERCISE	TEMPO	SETS	REPS	REST	WEIGHT (LBS)
A1) Split Squat/ Bulgarian Split Squat	3-0-1-0	3	10–12	30 seconds	
A2) Lat Pulldown/ Chin-up	3-0-1-0	3	10–12/ 8–10	60 seconds	
B1) Squat (Goblet/ Back)/ Front Squat	4-0-1-0	3	10–12	30 seconds	
B2) Dumbbell Row/ Barbell Row	3-0-1-1	3	10–12	60 seconds	
C1) Step-up/Barbell Step-up	2-0-1-0	3	12–15	30 seconds	
C2) Body-Weight Row/ Face Pull with Rope	3-0-1-1	3	10–12	60 seconds	

STRENGTH-TRAINING SESSION, DAY 3					
EXERCISE	TEMPO	SETS	REPS	REST	WEIGHT (LBS)
A1) Neutral Grip Lying Tricep Extension (Skull Crusher)/Tricep Extension with Rope	3-0-1-1	3	10–12	30 seconds	
A2) Bicep Curl/Incline Bench Dumbbell Curl	3-0-1-1	3	10–12	30 seconds	
B1) Thruster (Squat into Press)/Bicep Curl into Shoulder Press	3-0-1-0	3	10–12	60 seconds	
B2) Trap 3 Raise/ Dumbbell Snatch	2-0-1-0	3	10–12	30 seconds	
C1) Burpee/ Kettle Bell Swing	Constant Speed	3	10–12/ 20–25	30 seconds	
C2) Lying Twist (Windshield Wiper)/ Leg Lift or Knee Tuck	3-0-1-0	3	10–12 reps per side	60 seconds	

I have now given you all the bits and pieces of the Hormone Boost that you need to start living your new lifestyle. I'd like to leave you with a quotation I first shared in *The Hormone Diet* and still find fitting. It sums up perfectly the truly uncomplicated things we need to do daily—the benefits of which have been reinforced by the latest research and reported in these pages. Perhaps there is only one basic thing missing—play in the dirt and go barefoot (a process called "grounding," which has also been proven beneficial for us).

Live in rooms full of light
Avoid heavy food
Be moderate in the drinking of wine
Take massage, baths, exercise, and gymnastics
Fight insomnia with gentle rocking or the sound of running water
Change surroundings and take long journeys
Strictly avoid frightening ideas
Indulge in cheerful conversation and amusements
Listen to music.

AULUS CORNELIUS CELSUS,
Roman encyclopedist, ca. 25 BC–ca. AD 50

If embarking on the complete Hormone Boost feels daunting, remember that you have the rest of your life to be healthy! Start with the simple steps, if nothing else, and add in one new thing each week. I love the following words from Henry Ford; house them in your mind to sustain you: "When everything seems to be going against you, remember that the airplane takes off against the wind, not with it." Happy Boosting!

PART FOUR

FOOD LISTS, SHOPPING LISTS AND RECIPES

A successful man is one who can lay a firm foundation with the bricks others have thrown at him.

DAVID BRINKLEY,
American newscaster for NBC and ABC from 1943 to 1997

CHAPTER 13

PERMITTED FOODS AND GROCERY LISTS

Now that you have the Hormone Boost theory, science and framework under your belt, you're set to discover and experience the great-tasting foods that make up this simple, fast-acting diet. I've made it easy for you to get started by creating lists of foods to enjoy and to avoid, meals and even shopping lists.

To create your own perfectly balanced Hormone Boost meals, you'll simply choose one protein, one carb, one fat and one fiber for each meal, four times a day, from the list of Foods to Enjoy. Unlike protein, fat or fiber, which have only one category on the list, there are three types of carbs: Green Vegetables, Fruits and Starchy Carbs. Select Green Vegetables for two to three meals each day, Fruits as your carb source for one (maximum two) meal(s) and a Starchy Carb for your evening meal selection (meal 4).

There are three food lists:

- one for the overall Hormone Boost diet plan
- one for Hormone Boost smoothies
- one for Hormone Boost salads

FOOD LISTS AND SERVING SIZES

Pick a Protein, Carb, Fat and Fiber to create your own Hormone Boost meal.

WOMEN: NUTRITIONAL GUIDELINES PER MEAL	MEN: NUTRITIONAL GUIDELINES PER MEAL
Protein: 25–35 g	Protein: 35–45 g
Carbs: 20–30 g	Carbs: 30–40 g
Fats: 10–14 g	Fats: 14–18 g
Fiber: 4–10 g	Fiber: 4–10 g

FOODS TO ENJOY AND SUGGESTED SERVING SIZES		FOODS TO AVOID
PROTEINS (NOTE: The first number listed after the food is the suggested serving size, while the number in brackets is the amount of protein in that serving. So 5 oz. of lean red meat contains 28 to 33 g of protein. Four to 5 oz. of meat is about the size and width of the area from the edge of your palm to the middle knuckle.)		PROTEINS
Lean red meat (preferably organic, grass-fed)	5 oz. (28–33 g)	ALWAYS AVOID:
Chicken	4–5 oz. (30 g)	Luncheon meats or cold cuts that contain nitrates and sulfites
Turkey	4–5 oz. (30 g)	Sausages (those from a natural or local butcher are usually okay)
Shrimp	4–5 medium	Bacon
Scallop	3 large or 4 medium	Marbled meats
Crab	4 oz.	Deep-fried foods
Lobster (rock)	1	LIMIT:
Lobster tail	1 (39 g)	Tofu (tempeh is a better option)
Egg whites	2/3 cup (or 4–5 egg whites)	

FOODS TO ENJOY AND SUGGESTED SERVING SIZES		FOODS TO AVOID
Eggs	2 whole eggs plus 2 whites, or 3 egg whites and 1 whole egg with an additional fat source	
Tempeh	8 oz.	
Cottage cheese, ricotta cheese	1¼ cups (30 g)	
Organic pressed cottage cheese	½ cup (30 g)	
Allégro 4% cheese (try the jalapeno or herb flavor)	3 servings (33 g)	
Liberté Greek yogurt (0% or 2%)	1 serving (20 g)	
Liberté organic yogurt (plain, low-fat or no-fat)	¾ cup (13 g)	
Goat-milk yogurt (plain)	(8–10 g)	
Sheep-milk Greek yogurt	(8–10 g)	
Water buffalo yogurt	(8–10 g)	
Goat cheese, sheep cheese (could be more of a fat source)	serving size will vary	
PROTEIN BARS AND PROTEIN SUPPLEMENTS (NOTE: All selections must be free of sugar and artificial sweeteners.)		PROTEIN BARS AND PROTEIN SUPPLEMENTS
Whey protein powder (my favorite brand is Dream Protein)	1 scoop (20 g)	ALWAYS AVOID:
Vegan protein powders such as rice, hemp or pea protein. Recommended brands include Vega One, Sunwarrior, PaleoMeal (Designs for Health) and Vegan Protein + (Genuine Health)		Soy protein powders
Ultra Protein Bar (Metagenics) (offers a complete meal source on the go)	1 bar (23 g)	Egg protein powders

FOODS TO ENJOY AND SUGGESTED SERVING SIZES		FOODS TO AVOID
Clear Complete meal replacement	1 scoop (16 g) (1.5–2 scoops offers a whey protein–based complete meal source on the go)	Any protein supplement containing sucralose or other artificial sweeteners
Clear Vegan – Protein Complete Cleanse	1 scoop (16 g)	
PaleoMeal DF (pea protein–based meal replacement)		Any protein bar or meal replacement that does not hit the macronutrient guidelines of the Hormone Boost
UltraMeal Bar Rice Protein	1 bar (12 g) (Chocolate Fudge flavor only—and even this one, which is the lowest in carbs, isn't as high in protein or as low in carbs as I would like)	Quest bars (contain GMO corn)
		Bars with harmful oils, sucralose or high carb or high fat content
Rumble Supershake	1 bottle (20 g) (a whey protein–based complete meal option on the go)	
B-UP bars	1 bar (20 g) (a whey protein–based complete meal option on the go)	
CARBS: Green Vegetables (Select Green Vegetables as your carb source for two to three meals each day—in the form of salads, raw, steamed, stir-fried or in soups. The suggested serving size is 2–3 cups when they are consumed as the sole carbohydrate source in a meal, and 1–2 cups when they are combined with a Starchy Carb or Fruit.)		CARBS: Vegetables
All green vegetables (broccoli, spinach, zucchini, Brussels sprouts, rapini, green beans, cucumber, etc.)		AVOID (except for your cheat meal, once a week):
Peppers		White and sweet potatoes
Tomatoes		Corn
Eggplant		Parsnips
Cauliflower		

FOODS TO ENJOY AND SUGGESTED SERVING SIZES		FOODS TO AVOID
Onions		
Leeks		
Artichokes		
CARBS: Fruit (Select Fruit as your carb source for one to two meals each day. Berries and Asian pear are the best choices.)		CARBS: Fruit
Cherries	12	AVOID (except for your cheat meal, once a week):
Apricots	3	Melon (cantaloupe, honey-dew, etc.)
Prunes	3	Pineapple
Berries	½ cup	Papaya
Peach	1 small	Mango
Pear	1 small	Grapes
Apple	1 small	Dried fruit (except goji berries)
Plum	1	
Orange	1 small	
Kiwifruit	1 small	
Grapefruit	1 whole	
Watermelon	1 cup	
Banana	½ (in protein shakes only)	
Goji berries	2 tablespoons	
CARBS: Starchy (Select one serving each day for meal 4 only, about the size of your fist; ½ cup; or serving otherwise specified)		CARBS: Starchy
Carrots (cooked, raw or baby)	1 cup	AVOID (except for your cheat meal, once a week):
Soybeans/edamame (shelled)	1 cup	White bread
Summer squash	1 cup	White pasta
Beets (sliced)	1 cup	Bagels
Celery root (celeriac)	1 cup	Muffins

FOODS TO ENJOY AND SUGGESTED SERVING SIZES		FOODS TO AVOID
Peas (green)	1 cup	Pastries and pies
Winter squash (acorn or butternut)	1 cup	Cookies
Water chestnuts	1 cup	Any product labeled "energy bar"
Calico beans		Spelt products
Broad beans (fava beans)		Crackers
Lentils		Granola bars
Split peas		Sesame snacks
Great Northern beans		Oatmeal
Mung beans		Whole-wheat products
Black beans		Brown rice
Butter beans		Kamut bread or pasta
Kidney beans		Hummus
Cannellini beans (white kidney beans)		Chickpeas
Navy beans		
Lima beans		
Pinto beans		
Rye bread (brands that are low carb, like Dimpflmeier Dark Rye)		
Udi's Millet-Chia Bread	1–2 slices	
Ezekiel Bread	1–2 slices	
Gluten-free wraps, like those made with coconut flour (e.g., Pure Wraps)		
Mary's crackers	13 crackers	
Bulgur		
Buckwheat groats/kasha		
Quinoa		
Oat bran		
FATS		FATS

FOODS TO ENJOY AND SUGGESTED SERVING SIZES		FOODS TO AVOID
Olive oil (recommended daily)	1 tablespoon	ALWAYS AVOID:
Avocado	¼	Hydrogenated oils and trans fatty acids
Mayonnaise (canola- or olive-oil based)	1 tablespoon	Palm oil
Olives	6	Flaxseed oil
Butter (grass-fed is best)	1 teaspoon	Soy oil
Omega-3 egg yolks	2–3	Corn oil
Organic coconut butter or oil	1 tablespoon	Cottonseed oil
Salad dressings made with canola or olive oil	1 tablespoon	Vegetable oil
Walnuts	16	Shortening
Cashews	12	Margarine
Almonds	15–20	Peanuts and peanut butter (if you do have them, they must be organic)
Pistachios	40–50	LIMIT:
Seeds (pumpkin, sunflower or sesame)	2 tablespoons	Safflower oil
Nut butter (cashew, macadamia, almond or pumpkin seed)	1 tablespoon	Sunflower oil
Hemp seeds	2 tablespoons	
FIBER (NOTE: Chia seeds and flax seeds are best to sprinkle on meals and salads, while a fiber supplement is best for smoothies because it provides double the amount of fiber per serving. Chia seeds and flax seeds alone will not meet your fiber needs.)		
Chia seeds	2 tablespoons (4 g)	
Flax seeds	2 tablespoons (4 g)	
Solufiber (AOR)	10 g	
Clear Fiber	8 g	
Fiber supplement from health food store		

FOODS TO ENJOY AND SUGGESTED SERVING SIZES		FOODS TO AVOID
Herbulk (Metagenics) (better suited for those prone to loose stools)	8 g	
UltraProtein Bar (Metagenics)	10 g (complete meal option on the go)	
Clear Complete meal replacement	1 scoop (8 g) (complete meal option on the go)	
Rumble Supershake	1 bottle (6 g) (complete meal option on the go)	
UltraMeal Bar Rice Protein	1 bar (6 g) (Chocolate Fudge flavor only—and even this one, which is the lowest in carbs, isn't as high in protein or as low in carbs as I would like)	
B-UP bar	1 bar (20 g)	
SPICES AND CONDIMENTS		SPICES AND CONDIMENTS
All spices and herbs unless otherwise indicated (e.g., cinnamon, cumin, dill, garlic, ginger, carob, oregano, parsley, rosemary, tarragon, thyme, turmeric, etc.)		AVOID (except for your cheat meal, once a week):
Mustard		Ketchup
Xyla ketchup and barbecue sauce		Relish
Low-carb salad dressings made with olive or canola oil		Pickles
		Chutney
		Soy sauce
		Barbecue sauce or other condiments containing sugar

FOODS TO ENJOY AND SUGGESTED SERVING SIZES	FOODS TO AVOID
DRINKS	FOODS OR DRINKS CONTAINING:
Sodium-free soda water	Sugar (except for your cheat meal once a week)
All herbal teas	Alcohol (you may have two to four drinks per week. Red wine is preferred, but if you suspect yeast overgrowth is an issue, drink only vodka, gin or tequila.)
Reverse-osmosis water is preferred	
Pure fruit juices should be limited to smoothies or mixed with water ($^1/_4$ cup juice to $^3/_4$ cup water or sparkling water)	
Organic coffee (with cream or whipping cream, before noon, without sugar or sweeteners; add cinnamon if you like)	
Almond milk	
Cashew milk	
Coconut milk (from a carton)	
Bragg's Apple Cider Vinegar Drink Concord grape juice	

PICK-4 SALAD INGREDIENT LIST

Pick a Carb, Protein, Fat and Fiber to make your own Hormone Boost salad.

WOMEN: NUTRITIONAL GUIDELINES PER SALAD	MEN: NUTRITIONAL GUIDELINES PER SALAD
Carbs: 20–30 g	Carbs: 30–40 g
Protein: 25–35 g	Protein: 35–45 g
Fats: 10–14 g	Fats: 14–18 g
Fiber: 4–10 g	Fiber: 4–10 g

FOODS TO ENJOY	FOODS TO AVOID
CARBS: Greens (The suggested serving size is 2–3 cups.)	
Kale	
Baby spinach	
Beet greens	
Broccoli	
Swiss chard	
Arugula	
Broccoli sprouts	
Endive (frisée)	
Radicchio	
Escarole	
Watercress	
Bok choy	
Romaine	
Butter lettuce	
Field lettuce	
Green or red leaf lettuce	

FOODS TO ENJOY	FOODS TO AVOID
CARBS: Other Veggies (Note: These are optional. The suggested serving size for each is $\frac{1}{2}$ cup, or use $\frac{1}{4}$ cup maximum if you choose two or three options.)	CARBS: Other Veggies
Zucchini	AVOID (except for your cheat meal, once a week):
Red, yellow, orange and green peppers	White and sweet potatoes
Artichoke hearts	Corn
Hearts of palm	Parsnips
Mushrooms	
White onion	
Spanish onion	
Shallots	
Green onions	
Leeks	
Jicama	
Cabbage	
Cauliflower, broccoli, Brussels sprouts (steamed to reduce bloating effect)	
Radishes	
Snap peas	
Green and yellow beans	
Cucumber	
CARBS: Starchy (Select one serving each day at meal 4 only. The suggested serving size for each is $\frac{1}{2}$ cup unless otherwise stated, or use half or a third of the serving size if you choose two or three options.)	CARBS: Starchy
Carrots (grated, sliced, raw or cooked) 1 cup	AVOID (except for your cheat meal, once a week):
Edamame 1 cup	White bread
Summer squash 1 cup	White pasta
Beets (sliced) 1 cup	Spelt products
Celery root (celeriac) 1 cup	Crackers
Peas (green) 1 cup	Granola bars

FOODS TO ENJOY		FOODS TO AVOID
Winter squash (acorn or butternut)	1 cup	Sesame snacks
Water chestnuts		Oatmeal
Calico beans		Whole-wheat products
Broad beans (fava beans)		Brown rice
Lentils		Kamut bread or pasta
Split peas		Hummus
Great Northern beans		Chickpeas
Mung beans		
Black beans		
Butter beans		
Kidney beans		
Cannellini beans (white kidney beans)		
Navy beans		
Lima beans		
Pinto beans		
Bulgur		
Buckwheat groats/kasha		
Quinoa		
CARBS: Fruit (NOTE: Fruit is optional. Add one selection to your salad, or reduce serving sizes if you use two or three choices.)		CARBS: Fruit
Cherries	6	AVOID (except for your cheat meal, once a week):
Apricots (chopped)	2	Melon (cantaloupe, honeydew, etc.)
Prunes	2	Pineapple
Berries	1/4 cup	Papaya
Peach	1/2 small	Mango
Pear	1/2 small	Grapes
Apple	1/2 small	Dried fruit (except prunes and goji berries)
Plum	1	
Orange	1/2 small	

FOODS TO ENJOY		FOODS TO AVOID
Kiwifruit	1 small	
Grapefruit	½	
Watermelon	½ cup	
Goji berries	1 tablespoon	
Cherry tomatoes	6–8	
PROTEINS (Add one selection to your salad, or reduce serving sizes if you use two or three choices.)		**PROTEINS**
Lean red meat (preferably organic, grass-fed)	5 oz.	ALWAYS AVOID:
Chicken	4–5 oz.	Luncheon meats or cold cuts that contain nitrates and sulfites
Turkey	4–5 oz.	Sausages (those from a natural or local butcher are usually okay)
Shrimp	4 medium	Bacon
Scallops	3 large or 4 medium	Marbled meats
Crab	4 oz.	Deep-fried foods
Rock lobster	1 tail	Tofu
Fish (fresh or canned salmon or tuna; light is lowest in mercury)	1 can	
Egg whites	4	
Eggs	2–3 whole (remember the yolk adds fat)	
Tempeh	8 oz.	
Cottage cheese, ricotta cheese	¾–1 cup	
Organic pressed cottage cheese	½ cup	
Allégro 4% cheese (try the jalapeno or herb flavor)	3 servings (33 g)	
Goat cheese	sources vary in protein; keep an eye on fat content	

FOODS TO ENJOY		FOODS TO AVOID
Sheep cheese	sources vary in protein; keep an eye on fat content	
FATS (Add one selection to your salad, or reduce serving sizes if you use two or three choices.)		**FATS**
Olive oil	1 tablespoon	ALWAYS AVOID:
Avocado	$^1/_8$–$^1/_4$	Hydrogenated oils and trans fatty acids
Organic coconut butter or oil	1 tablespoon	Palm oil
Walnuts	16	Flaxseed oil
Cashews	12	Soy oil
Almonds	18	Corn oil
Pistachios	25–40	Cottonseed oil
Seeds (pumpkin, sunflower or sesame)	2 tablespoons	Vegetable oil
Nut butter (cashew, macadamia, almond or pumpkin seed)	1 tablespoon	Peanuts and peanut butter (if you do have them, they must be organic)
Hemp seeds	2 tablespoons	Shortening
My fave salad mix: pumpkin seeds with black and white sesame seeds, toasted (without oil), with Celtic sea salt	2 tablespoons	Margarines
		LIMIT:
		Safflower oil
		Sunflower oil
FIBER (Add one selection or a mixture of both. The serving size is 2 tablespoons.)		
Chia seeds		
Flax seeds		

FOODS TO ENJOY		FOODS TO AVOID
DRESSING BASE OPTIONS (The serving sizes are unlimited unless otherwise stated.)		
Lemon juice		
Apple cider vinegar		
Balsamic vinegar (choose an option low in sugar)	$^1/_4$ cup maximum	
White balsamic vinegar		
Rice wine vinegar		
Greek yogurt	1–2 tablespoons	
Yogurt	1–2 tablespoons	
Honey	1 teaspoon maximum if needed to sweeten dressing, or 1 teaspoon coconut sugar	
HERBS AND SPICES (Use these in unlimited quantities.)		
Dijon mustard		
Celtic sea salt		
Fresh black pepper		
Ginger		
Garlic (powder or bulb)		
Rosemary		
Dill		
Mrs. Dash		
Herbamare Sea Salt and Spice Mix		
Basil		
Oregano		
Thyme		

PICK-4 SMOOTHIE INGREDIENT LIST

Pick a Carb, Protein, Fat and Fiber to make up your own Hormone Boost smoothie.

WOMEN: NUTRITIONAL GUIDELINES PER SMOOTHIE	MEN: NUTRITIONAL GUIDELINES PER SMOOTHIE
Carbs: 20–30 g	Carbs: 30–40 g
Protein: 25–35 g	Protein: 35–45 g
Fats: 10–14 g	Fats: 14–18 g
Fiber: 4–10 g	Fiber: 4–10 g

FOODS TO ENJOY		FOODS TO AVOID
CARBS: Greens (The suggested serving size is about ½–1 cup. Use ½ cup if you are adding a fruit.)		
Kale		
Baby spinach		
Beet greens		
Broccoli		
Swiss chard		
Arugula		
Broccoli sprouts		
CARBS: Fruit (NOTE: Fruit is optional, but you may add one selection to your smoothie.)		CARBS: Fruit
Cherries	12	AVOID (except in post-workout smoothies):
Apricots	3	Melon (cantaloupe, honey-dew, etc.)
Prunes	3	Pineapple
Berries	½ cup	Papaya
Peach	1 small	Mango
Pear	1 small	Grapes
Apple	1 small	ALWAYS AVOID:
Plum	1	Dried fruit (except prunes and goji berries)

FOODS TO ENJOY		FOODS TO AVOID
Orange	1 small	
Kiwi	1 small	
Grapefruit	1 whole	
Watermelon	1 cup	
Banana	1/3–1/2, preferably frozen	
Goji berries	2 tablespoons	
PROTEINS (Add one selection to your smoothie. The first number listed after the food is the suggested serving size, while the number in brackets is the amount of protein in that serving. Note: Blend all the smoothie ingredients together except the protein, then add the protein and blend again briefly.)		**PROTEINS**
Liberté or Fage Greek yogurt (0% or 2%)	¾ cup (20 g)	AVOID:
Liberté or Fage Organic plain, low-fat or no-fat yogurt	¾ cup (20 g)	Soy protein powders (I prefer that you eat the whole-food soy source rather than a protein powder supplement)
Goat yogurt, plain (watch the fat content)	¾ cup (8–10 g)	Egg protein powder (I prefer that you eat the whole food)
Sheep Greek yogurt, plain (watch the fat content)	¾ cup (8–10 g)	Flavored yogurts
Water buffalo yogurt, plain	¾ cup (8–10 g)	Any protein powder containing artificial sweeteners
Clear Complete	1–2 scoops (offers a complete meal source on the go), or blend with an additional fat source but do not add any other carbs (i.e., fruit)	Hydrolysate proteins
Whey protein		
Vegan protein powders (such as rice, hemp or pea protein). Recommended brands include:		

FOODS TO ENJOY		FOODS TO AVOID
Clear Vegan – Protein Complete Cleanse	1 scoop (16 g protein, 8 g fiber)	
Sunwarrior	1–3 scoops, depending on the product	
Genuine Health Vegan Protein Powder	2 scoops (24 g)	
FATS (Add one selection to your smoothie.)		**FATS**
Olive oil	1 tablespoon	**ALWAYS AVOID:**
Avocado	$^1/_8$–$^1/_4$	Flaxseed oil
Organic coconut butter or oil	1 tablespoon	Peanuts and peanut butter (if you do have them, they must be organic)
Walnuts	16	
Cashews	12	
Almonds	18	
Pistachios	25–50	
Seeds (pumpkin, sunflower or sesame)	2 tablespoons	
Nut butter (cashew, macadamia, almond or pumpkin seed)	2 tablespoons	
Hemp seeds	2 tablespoons	
FIBER (Add one selection to your smoothie. Note: Chia seeds and flax seeds are best to sprinkle on meals and salads, while a fiber supplement is best for smoothies because it provides double the amount of fiber per serving. Chia seeds and flax seeds alone will not meet your fiber needs.)		**FIBER**
Solufiber (AOR)	10 g	Psyllium fiber may cause abdominal bloating or irritation. Choose an alternative source if you suspect this may be an issue for you.
Clear Fiber	8 g	
Herbulk (Metagenics)	8 g	
Chia seeds	2 tablespoons (4 g)	
Flax seeds	2 tablespoons (4 g)	

FOODS TO ENJOY		FOODS TO AVOID
LIQUID BASE OPTIONS ($^1/_2$ cup to 1 cup— your preference)		**LIQUID BASE OPTIONS**
Almond milk (best low-carb option)		**ALWAYS AVOID:**
Water (best low-carb option)		Cow's milk
Coconut water		Any sweetened milk products
Coconut milk (from a carton)		Any liquid containing artificial sweeteners
Cashew milk		
Soy milk (organic only)		
Rice milk		
Pure fruit juices (no more than $^1/_4$ cup juice mixed with $^3/_4$ cup water)		
Organic coffee (brewed or instant)		
Peppermint tea		
HERBS AND SPICES (Use these in unlimited quantities.)		
Fresh basil		
Fresh mint		
Fresh parsley		
Vanilla extract		
Vanilla bean		
Cinnamon		
Nutmeg		
Ginger		
Cloves		
Turmeric		
Celtic sea salt		
MEAL REPLACEMENTS (Protein, Carb, Fat and Fiber)		**MEAL REPLACEMENTS**
B-UP bar	1 bar (20 g fiber, 20 g whey protein)	Any protein bar or meal replacement that does not hit the macronutrient guidelines of the Hormone Boost
UltraProtein Bar (Metagenics)	(10 g fiber, 28 g protein)	Quest Bars (contain GMO corn)

FOODS TO ENJOY		FOODS TO AVOID
Clear Complete	1 scoop (6 g fiber, 18 g protein)	Bars with harmful oils, sucralose or high-carb content
Rumble Supershake	1 bottle (6 g fiber, 20 g protein)	
Clear Vegan – Protein Complete Cleanse	1 scoop (8 g fiber, 16 g protein)	

A Special Note for Vegans and Vegetarians

The challenge with diets like the Hormone Boost is that your available vegetable-based protein sources tend to be high in carbohydrates. Most of these foods also fail to provide enough protein to allow for the desired metabolic and hormonal benefits. Although several foods may commonly come to mind as go-to protein sources for vegetarians, the number containing a decent dose of this essential macronutrient, without the presence of too many carbs, is actually quite limited (as seen in the following chart). Most of you will benefit from using one or two of the sources listed in the chart combined with two different types of protein powders to hit your daily protein intake needs.

VEGETARIAN PROTEIN SOURCES

FOOD AND SERVING SIZE	PROTEIN (G)	CARB (G)	FIBER (G)
Tempeh – 1 cup	31	15.6	0
Seitan – 3 oz.	11	10	1
Soybeans, cooked – ½ cup	15	8	5
Lentils, cooked – ½ cup	9	20	9
Veggie burgers – 1 patty (nutrition content varies widely between brands)	10	9	3
Tofu – ½ cup	10	2	1
Textured vegetable protein – ½ cup cooked	24	14	8

Suggested Grocery Shopping Lists

Stocking the pantry doesn't have to be an overwhelming prospect. Here's a list of healthy, hormone-boosting foods to stock up on when you're ready to start your boost:

Dairy
Allégro 4% cheese
Goat cheese
Greek yogurt, 2% or 0%
Ricotta cheese

Spices, Herbs and Condiments
Balsamic vinegar
Basil (fresh and dried)
Bay leaves
Black pepper
Cajun seasoning (no salt added)
Capers
Cayenne
Celery salt
Chili powder
Cinnamon
Cloves (ground)
Cooking sherry
Coriander
Cumin
Curry powder
Dijon mustard
Dried oregano
Fresh dill, thyme, rosemary, cilantro, chives, parsley, tarragon
Garam masala
Garlic powder
Ginger root
Italian seasoning
Low-sodium chicken, beef and vegetable stock
Mrs. Dash Original Blend
Nutmeg
Organic honey (unpasteurized)
Red pepper flakes
Red wine vinegar
Rice wine vinegar
Salsa (no sugar added)
Sea salt
Smoked paprika
Tamari soy sauce (gluten-free)
Tomato paste
Turmeric
White wine vinegar

Oils/Nut Butters/Healthy Fats
Almond or cashew butter
Avocado
Coconut oil
Extra-virgin olive oil
Hemp seeds
Olive oil–based mayonnaise
Butter or ghee (preferably grass-fed, organic)
Organic olive oil spray
Sesame oil

Grain Substitutes
Almond flour
Brown or white basmati rice
Coconut flour
Quinoa

Nuts and Seeds (preferably raw and unsalted)
Almonds
Cashews
Chia seeds
Flax seeds
Pecans
Pistachios
Pumpkin seeds
Walnuts

Proteins (preferably natural, grass-fed and/ or organic)
Alaskan cod
Beef
Beef chuck roast
Chicken and turkey sausages
Chicken breast, boneless and skinless
Flank and sirloin steak
Free-range eggs
Ground turkey
Halibut
Salmon
Sea scallops
Shrimp
Sole
Tuna (canned, light)
Turkey bacon

Vegetables
Arugula
Asparagus
Bell peppers (red, yellow, orange)
Broccoli
Brown or green lentils (organic, canned)
Button mushrooms
Cannellini beans (organic canned)
Carrots

Cauliflower
Celery
Coleslaw mix
Crushed tomatoes
(organic, canned, no
salt added)
Cucumber
Garlic
Kale

Lettuce (romaine or
Boston)
Onions (white, Spanish,
green or shallots)
Pumpkin purée (organic,
canned)
Radishes
Rapini
Red potatoes

Roma tomatoes (organic,
canned, no salt added)
Shallots
Spaghetti squash
Spinach
Sun dried tomatoes
Swiss chard
Tomatoes (fresh Roma or
cherry)
Zucchini

Smoothie Shopping List

Fruits (frozen or fresh,
preferably organic)
Bananas (I recommend
cutting them in half or
thirds and freezing)
Berries (blackberries,
raspberries, strawber-
ries, blueberries or a
frozen berry blend)
Cherries (tart)
Peaches
Pears
Royal Gala apples

**Greens and Vegetables
(preferably organic)**
Baby kale
Baby spinach
Pumpkin purée (canned)

**Herbs, Spices and
Extracts**
Basil, fresh

Celtic sea salt
Cinnamon
Cloves
Ginger
Mint, fresh
Nutmeg
Turmeric
Vanilla bean
Vanilla extract

Liquids
Cashew or almond milk
Coconut milk (in a carton)
Coffee (instant or brewed)
Peppermint tea

Protein
Greek yogurt, 0% or 2%
fat content, plain
Protein powder (whey,
rice, hemp, pea or
another vegan option)

Fats
Almond butter
Avocado (I recommend
slicing it into quarters
and freezing)
Cashew butter
Cashews
Coconut oil
Hazelnut butter
Hemp seeds
Walnuts

Fiber
Chia seeds
Fiber supplement
Flax seeds

Other Items
Cacao powder
Cacao nibs
Matcha green tea powder
Spirulina

CHAPTER 14

THE RECIPES

Now for the fun part! I have included more than 50 recipes in this book, and I encourage you to try as many of these delicious meals as you can. Honestly, I think these are my best recipes yet! And I've made sure you can customize everything to your tastes; just use the food lists in Chapter 13 to alter any ingredients that do not appeal to you. For instance, if a recipe calls for cashews and you don't like cashews, simply find them on the list and choose any other item in that category as a replacement.

Each recipe includes nutrition information. Naturally, the exact content will vary depending on the food source or product selection, but the numbers should help you stick pretty closely to the macronutrient guidelines of the Hormone Boost. Protein, carb, fat and fiber content are listed, but you'll notice that I've left out the calorie count. This is because the *source* of your calories is a more important marker for hormonal balance.

Grab-and-Go Meal Ideas

Yes, you're about to be introduced to a bunch of delicious recipes to keep you inspired, satisfied and on track. But let's face it, there are days when you just don't have time to putter in the kitchen. What happens then? The following is a list of ideas that require little to no cooking time.

Carb-Free Meal 1:

- 1.5 to 2 scoops of Clear Complete plus 1 to 2 tablespoons of hemp seeds; shake or blend with one of the permitted liquid bases and ice
- 1 to 2 (depending on the size) turkey or chicken sausages and 1 serving of cashews (or any other nut)
- Chicken burger topped with guacamole (such as the frozen all-natural option from Costco)
- 2 eggs and 2 egg whites scrambled with salsa and goat cheese
- 2 to 3 boiled eggs

Meals 2 and 3:

- Any salad created using the Hormone Boost Pick-4 Salad Ingredient List (page 254)
- Any smoothie created using the Hormone Boost Pick-4 Smoothie Ingredient List (page 260)
- A healthy premade vegetable or legume (such as lentil or black bean) soup option (carb-conscious and free of additives), or a previously prepped serving of homemade soup (cook or purée veggies, ginger, carrots, onion, 1/2 cup of cooked beans, 1 tablespoon of olive oil, water and desired spices). Add 4 to 5 ounces of a lean protein source or enjoy the protein, grilled or baked, on the side, or top with 3/4 to 1 cup of ricotta or pressed organic cottage cheese
- Vegetable curry with tempeh or sliced chicken breast (no rice)
- 2 whole eggs (but skip one yolk) plus diced veggies, fresh herbs or spices and about 1 tablespoon of goat cheese (or enjoy 2 whole eggs and skip the goat cheese)
- Greek yogurt with 1/2 cup of berries, 2 tablespoons ground flax or chia seeds and 2 tablespoons hemp seeds or 1 serving of nuts

- Greek yogurt with 1 teaspoon of hemp seeds and 15 almonds
- 1 scoop of any of my suggested protein powders and 1 scoop of Clear Recovery (my post-workout strength and energy formula) in water
- Any permitted protein bar or protein meal replacement (limit yourself to no more than one protein bar per day)

Quick and Easy
(Options to Make Ahead and Consume on the Go)

PROTEIN PANCAKES (STARCHY CARB–FREE/ON THE GO)
Serves 4

½ banana
¼ avocado
3 egg whites
2 tablespoons vanilla almond or coconut milk (from carton)
1 serving vanilla protein powder
½–1 teaspoon cinnamon
1 packet stevia (optional)
Coconut oil cooking spray

In a medium-sized bowl, mash the banana and avocado together until smooth. Stir in the egg whites, vanilla almond milk, vanilla protein powder, cinnamon and stevia (if using). Lightly grease a skillet with cooking spray and place over medium-high heat. Pour batter into four rounds in the pan, spreading it out with a spatula if needed. Cook the pancakes for 1 to 2 minutes, turning them over once or twice, until they are firm. Serve the pancakes topped with Greek yogurt, or spread with almond butter and roll up for a portable breakfast.

Protein: 35 g | Carb: 25.3 g | Fat: 10.6 g | Fiber: 7 g

ZUCCHINI PANCAKES (STARCHY CARB–FREE/ON THE GO)
Serves 3–4

8 eggs

2 tablespoons coconut flour

Sea salt and pepper to taste

4 cups shredded zucchini

Olive oil or coconut oil cooking spray

2 cups plain 2% Greek yogurt

In a large bowl, whisk the eggs together with the coconut flour, sea salt and pepper. Stir in the shredded zucchini; mix well. Lightly grease a skillet with cooking spray and place over low heat. Using 1 heaping tablespoon of batter for each pancake, cook the pancakes until golden brown on one side, then flip and cook on the other side. Remove from the pan and top each serving with $\frac{1}{2}$ cup of Greek yogurt.

Protein: 27 g | Carb: 13 g | Fat: 16 g | Fiber: 3 g

SPINACH-MUSHROOM CRUSTLESS QUICHE CUPS (STARCHY CARB–FREE/ON THE GO)
Serves 6–8

1 tablespoon extra-virgin olive oil

2 cups sliced button mushrooms

1 yellow onion, diced

1 package (10 ounces) fresh spinach

$\frac{1}{4}$ cup water

8 eggs

1 cup shredded Allégro 4% cheese (optional)

Sea salt and pepper to taste

Preheat the oven to 375°F. In a large skillet, heat the oil over medium heat. Add the mushrooms and onion and sauté until softened and liquid is evaporated, 5 to 6 minutes. Set aside on a plate. Add the spinach and water to the skillet and cook just until wilted, 3 to 4 minutes. Remove from the heat.

In a large mixing bowl, whisk the eggs until combined. Add the cooked mushrooms and onion, spinach, cheese (if using) and salt and pepper. Divide evenly among 6 to 8 greased muffin cups. Bake for 20 to 23 minutes or until well set and a toothpick inserted in the center comes out clean. Let sit for a few minutes or until the pan is cool enough to handle. Sprinkle with a little more cheese and salt and pepper, if desired.

Protein: 17 g | Carb: 4.7 g | Fat: 12.9 g | Fiber: 1.9 g

QUICK AND EASY MASON JAR SALAD (STARCHY CARB–FREE/ ON THE GO)
Serves 1
The chicken in this recipe can be replaced with a vegan protein source such as tempeh, or with another protein from the Foods to Enjoy list. You can substitute spinach or kale for the mixed greens, making for endless lunch possibilities.

2 tablespoons extra-virgin olive oil
4 tablespoons rice wine vinegar
8 cherry tomatoes, halved
¼ cup diced cucumber
½ red bell pepper, diced
5 radishes, sliced
2 green onions, thinly sliced
¼ avocado
2 cups mixed greens
½ cup diced cooked chicken or turkey breast
¼ cup pumpkin seeds
Dried basil to taste
Pepper to taste

In a Mason jar, combine the olive oil and rice wine vinegar, then add the rest of the ingredients. Keep the jar upright until ready to serve, then shake it or use a fork to mix the ingredients together, and pour the salad into a dish.

Protein: 29.7 g | Carb: 29.9 g | Fat: 15.2 g | Fiber: 10.8 g

Meals 1, 2 and 3: Starchy Carb–Free Options

THAI TURKEY LETTUCE WRAPS (STARCHY CARB–FREE)
Serves 3

For an on-the-go lunch, pack the turkey mixture, lettuce leaves, carrots, bean sprouts and cilantro, and the drizzling sauce separately, and assemble the wraps when you are ready to eat.

2 teaspoons extra-virgin olive oil
12 ounces ground turkey
8 ounces button mushrooms, chopped
1 can (6 ounces) water chestnuts, drained and chopped
3 green onions, sliced
2 cloves garlic, minced
¼ cup gluten-free tamari soy sauce
1 tablespoon rice wine vinegar
2 teaspoons coconut sugar
9–12 large iceberg lettuce leaves
1 cup shredded carrots
1 cup bean sprouts
Fresh cilantro, chopped
Drizzling Sauce (recipe follows)

In a large skillet, heat the oil over medium-high heat. Add the turkey and cook until brown. Add the mushrooms, water chestnuts, green onions and garlic and sauté until the liquid has evaporated and the mushrooms are browned. In a small bowl, combine the soy sauce, rice wine vinegar and coconut sugar; pour over the turkey and vegetables and bring to a boil, stirring, until the sauce thickens.

Arrange 3 to 4 lettuce leaves on each plate. Spoon some turkey mixture into each leaf and top with shredded carrots, bean sprouts, cilantro and Drizzling Sauce.

DRIZZLING SAUCE
$\frac{1}{4}$ cup water
3 tablespoons gluten-free tamari soy sauce
2 tablespoons rice wine vinegar
1 tablespoon Dijon or spicy mustard
$1\frac{1}{2}$ teaspoons coconut sugar
1 teaspoon Sriracha sauce
$\frac{1}{2}$ teaspoon sesame oil

In a small bowl, whisk together all the ingredients. Set aside until ready to serve.

Protein: 28.4 g | Carb: 32.4 g | Fat: 14 g | Fiber: 3.5 g

LEMON TAMARI CHICKEN SALAD (STARCHY CARB–FREE)
Serves 2
Juice of 1 lemon
1 teaspoon gluten-free tamari soy sauce
1 teaspoon honey
1 teaspoon minced ginger root
$\frac{1}{2}$ teaspoon sea salt
1 tablespoon extra-virgin olive oil
2 tablespoons slivered raw almonds
1 tablespoon black and white sesame seeds
2 cooked boneless, skinless chicken breasts (4–5 ounces each), sliced
3 cups shredded cabbage

1 cup sugar snap peas

¼ cup sliced cucumber

In a small bowl, combine the lemon juice, soy sauce, honey, ginger and salt; gradually whisk in the oil. Add the slivered almonds and sesame seeds. In a large bowl, combine the chicken, cabbage, sugar snap peas and cucumber. Drizzle with the lemon juice mixture and toss.

Protein: 27 g | Carb: 19.8 g | Fat: 16 g | Fiber: 5 g

BAKED SALMON AND ASPARAGUS IN FOIL (STARCHY CARB–FREE)

Serves 4

2 pounds asparagus, trimmed

1 tablespoon extra-virgin olive oil

2 cloves garlic, minced

Sea salt and pepper to taste

4 skinless salmon fillets (4 ounces each)

Olive oil cooking spray

1 tablespoon chopped fresh dill, thyme or rosemary

1 lemon, thinly sliced

Preheat oven to 400°F. Cut four sheets of aluminum foil, each about 6 to 8 inches long. Divide the asparagus evenly among the sheets of foil. In a small bowl, stir together the olive oil and garlic; drizzle over each asparagus portion, then sprinkle with salt and pepper. Rinse the salmon and allow excess water to run off. Season the bottom of each fillet with salt and pepper and lay over the asparagus portions. Spray each fillet with cooking spray and season with salt and pepper; top with the fresh dill or herb of your choice and 2 lemon slices. Wrap the sides of the foil over the salmon, then fold over the ends to enclose the salmon. Place the foil pouches in a single layer on a baking sheet and bake 25 to 30 minutes, or until salmon is cooked through.

Protein: 25.2 g | Carb: 5.6 g | Fat: 14.9 g | Fiber: 4.8 g

RAINBOW THAI CHICKEN SALAD (STARCHY CARB–FREE)
Serves 2

2 cooked boneless, skinless chicken breasts (4–5 ounces each), sliced

2 cups shredded red cabbage

1 cup shredded green cabbage

1 large carrot, julienned or shredded

1 red bell pepper, julienned

1 cup chopped fresh cilantro

½ avocado, diced

½ cup chopped green onions

1 tablespoon sesame seeds, toasted

2 teaspoons sesame oil

DRESSING

2 tablespoons gluten-free tamari soy sauce

2 tablespoons rice wine vinegar

2–3 tablespoons hot water

1 tablespoon organic almond butter

Juice of 1 lime

1 teaspoon honey

Pinch red pepper flakes

DRESSING: In a small bowl, whisk all the dressing ingredients together until combined. If the dressing is too thick, add 1 teaspoon hot water at a time until the desired consistency is reached. Set aside.

In a salad bowl, toss together the chicken, red cabbage, green cabbage, carrot, bell pepper, cilantro, avocado, green onions, sesame seeds and sesame oil. Drizzle with dressing and toss again.

Protein: 32.6 g | Carb: 28.5 g | Fat: 15.1 g | Fiber: 2.7 g

SUNNY MEDITERRANEAN CHICKEN (STARCHY CARB–FREE)

Serves 2

1 tablespoon dried oregano

1 tablespoon smoked paprika

1–3 teaspoons, or to taste

1 teaspoon sea salt

Juice of 1 lemon or lime

2 boneless, skinless chicken breasts (4–5 ounces each)

3 bell peppers, assorted colors, chopped

2 jalapeno peppers, seeded and sliced

2 medium tomatoes, diced

2 small zucchini, diced

2 green onions, sliced

Preheat oven to 450°F. In a small bowl, combine the oregano, paprika, pepper, salt and lemon juice; spread over the chicken and place it in a small roasting pan or baking dish. Add both peppers, tomatoes, zucchini and green onions to the pan, and cover with aluminum foil. Bake for 35 minutes. Remove the foil, set the oven to broil and cook for an additional 5 minutes, or until the chicken is cooked through.

Protein: 29.5 g | Carb: 99.4 g | Fat: 8 g | Fiber: 4.9 g

COMFORTING ROSEMARY CHICKEN WITH SAUTÉED RAPINI (A.K.A. BROCCOLI RABE) (STARCHY CARB–FREE)

Serves 3

2 tablespoons extra-virgin olive oil, divided

3 boneless, skinless chicken breasts (4–5 ounces each)

Sea salt and pepper to taste

1 tablespoon unsalted butter

6 cloves garlic, thinly sliced, divided

3 sprigs fresh rosemary, chopped

1 bunch rapini, bottoms trimmed (but leave the full stalk on each piece)

4 small zucchini, cut into long strips
Juice of 1 lemon
Lemon slices

Preheat oven to 425° F. In an ovenproof skillet, heat 1 tablespoon of the oil over medium-high heat until the oil is hot. Add the chicken and season with salt and pepper. Sear the chicken until browned, about 4 minutes per side. Add the butter, half of the garlic, and the rosemary to the pan, and transfer to the oven to roast for 20 minutes, glazing with the garlic drippings if desired, until the chicken is cooked through.

While the chicken is in the oven, add the remaining oil and garlic to another skillet over medium heat. Add the rapini and a pinch of salt and cook until tender, about 8 to 10 minutes. Add the zucchini and cook until tender. Sprinkle with lemon juice. Divide the rapini and zucchini among three plates and top each with a chicken breast and a drizzle of garlic oil from the pan. Garnish with lemon slices.

Protein: 34.3 g | Carb: 10.7 g | Fat: 14.8 g | Fiber: 5.3 g

SASSY SPINACH SALAD WITH GRILLED CHICKEN (STARCHY CARB–FREE)
Serves 2
2 grilled boneless, skinless chicken breasts (4–5 ounces each), sliced
6 cups spinach
2 Roma tomatoes, cut in wedges
2 stalks celery, chopped
½ cucumber, thinly sliced
½ cup canned or bottled organic artichoke hearts, drained and chopped
¼ red onion, sliced
½ cup pumpkin seeds, toasted
½ to 1 teaspoon sea salt

DRESSING

3 tablespoons organic almond butter

3 tablespoons unsweetened almond or cashew milk

1 tablespoon honey

1 tablespoon Dijon or grainy mustard

Sea salt and pepper to taste

DRESSING: In a small bowl, whisk together all the dressing ingredients; set aside.

In a salad bowl, toss together the chicken, spinach, tomatoes, celery, cucumber, artichoke hearts, red onion, pumpkin seeds and sea salt. Drizzle with dressing and toss again.

Protein: 38.2 g | Carb: 33.7 g | Fat: 15.3 g | Fiber: 3.7 g

SEPHERHA'S CHICKEN FAJITA LETTUCE WRAPS
(STARCHY CARB–FREE)

Serves 4

You can substitute 3 servings of tempeh for the chicken in this recipe for a vegetarian meal.

3 tablespoons extra-virgin olive oil, divided

3 large boneless, skinless chicken breasts (about 6 ounces each), sliced

Chili powder, cumin, oregano, paprika, red pepper flakes and/or turmeric to taste

1 medium jar salsa (sugar-free)

8 cloves garlic, minced, divided

1 white onion, chopped

1 small zucchini, cut in strips

1 large red bell pepper, cut in strips

1 large yellow or orange bell pepper, cut in strips

1 head romaine or Boston lettuce, separated into leaves

AVOCADO CREMA

1 avocado

1 cup plain 0% Greek yogurt

3 tablespoons fresh lime juice

1/4 cup chopped fresh cilantro

1 to 2 cloves garlic, minced

PICO DE GALLO

2–3 large vine-ripened tomatoes, diced

1 white onion, diced

1 jalapeno pepper, minced

1 clove garlic, minced

3 tablespoons fresh lime juice

1/4 cup chopped fresh cilantro

AVOCADO CREMA: In the bowl of a food processor, combine the avocado, yogurt, lime juice, cilantro and the desired amount of garlic. Blend until smooth; set aside.

PICO DE GALLO: In a medium bowl, combine the tomatoes, onion, jalapeno, garlic, lime juice and cilantro; set aside.

In a large skillet, heat 1 tablespoon of the oil over medium-high heat. Add the chicken and sprinkle with the spices of your choice; stir-fry until the chicken is no longer pink. Add the salsa and 6 cloves of the garlic and cook until the chicken is cooked through; set aside.

In a separate skillet, heat 2 tablespoons of the oil over medium-low heat. Add the onion, zucchini, bell peppers, remaining 2 cloves of garlic, and the spices of your choice and cook for 5 minutes, until tender-crisp. Wrap the chicken mixture, vegetables, Avocado Crema and Pico de Gallo in lettuce leaves.

Protein: 26.7 g | Carb: 23.5 g | Fat: 13.5 g | Fiber: 3.9 g

JACKIE'S CHICKEN AND YOGURT CURRY (STARCHY CARB–FREE)
Serves 4

If you want to make this a Starchy Carb meal, have it with ½ cup of cooked quinoa per serving.

1 medium white onion, diced

1 tablespoon minced ginger root

4 cloves garlic, chopped

½ cup chopped fresh cilantro, plus more for garnish

2 tablespoons coconut oil

1 tablespoon turmeric (or more, to taste)

3 tablespoons garam masala

2 tablespoons curry powder

2 tablespoons cumin

½ teaspoon chili powder (optional)

½ teaspoon sea salt

1 cup plain 0% or 2% Greek yogurt

1 can (28 ounces) organic Roma tomatoes (no salt added)

16 ounces boneless, skinless chicken breasts, cubed

In the bowl of a food processor, combine the onion, ginger, garlic and cilantro and blend to a smooth paste; set aside. In a large skillet, heat the coconut oil over low heat. Add the onion mixture and sauté for 5 to 6 minutes. Add the turmeric, garam masala, curry powder, cumin, chili powder and salt and sauté for another 2 minutes. Stir in the yogurt, then add the tomatoes; simmer for 25 to 30 minutes, until the desired thickness is reached. Adjust seasonings to taste. Stir in the chicken and simmer gently for 10 to 15 minutes, until the chicken is cooked through. Garnish with cilantro.

Protein: 32 g | Carb: 14 g (without quinoa) 34 g (with quinoa) | Fat: 10.8 g | Fiber: 3 g

SPICY BASIL ZUCCHINI PASTA WITH PECAN-CRUSTED CHICKEN (STARCHY CARB–FREE)

Serves 4

½ cup almond meal or flour

4 pecans

2 tablespoons Mrs. Dash Original Blend

Sea salt and pepper to taste

1 egg, beaten

4 boneless, skinless chicken breasts (4–5 ounces each)

Zucchini Noodles (recipe follows)

Preheat oven to 400°F. In the bowl of a food processor, combine the almond meal, pecans, Mrs. Dash and salt and pepper, and pulse until the pecans are ground; set aside. In a bowl, whisk the egg. Dip each chicken breast into the egg and then dredge in the almond meal mixture, coating both sides, and place on a foil-lined baking sheet lightly greased with cooking spray. Bake for 20 to 25 minutes. Serve with Zucchini Noodles.

ZUCCHINI NOODLES

8 zucchini

Coconut oil cooking spray

PESTO

10 basil leaves

3 medium zucchini

Sliver of jalapeno pepper

Zest and juice of 1 lemon

¼ cup pecans, chopped

1 teaspoon coconut oil

Sea salt and pepper

Water, as needed

PESTO: In the bowl of a food processor, combine the basil, zucchini, jalapeno, lemon zest and juice, pecans, coconut oil and salt and pepper to taste; blend until finely chopped. With the motor running, add water through the feed tube until a smooth paste consistency is reached; set aside.

With a spiralizer, cut the zucchini into noodles. Lightly grease a large skillet with cooking spray and set over high heat. Add the zucchini noodles and sauté for 5 minutes. Remove from the heat and toss with the Pesto.

Protein: 32 g | Carb: 15 g | Fat: 13.1 g | Fiber: 2.9 g

DECONSTRUCTED COD TACO SALAD (STARCHY CARB–FREE)
Serves 2

2 chipotle peppers in adobo sauce (Herdez brand), minced, with 2 tablespoons of sauce
¼ cup finely chopped red onion
Juice of ½ lime
1 tablespoon extra-virgin olive oil
Sea salt to taste
2 Alaskan cod fillets (4 ounces each), cut into chunks
Coleslaw (recipe follows)
Fresh cilantro, chopped

In a large bowl, combine the chipotle peppers, adobo sauce, onion, lime juice, oil and a dash or two of salt. Add the fish and coat thoroughly. Cover and marinate in the fridge for a maximum of 20 minutes.

Preheat oven to 375°F. Cover a baking sheet with parchment paper. Place the marinated fish in one layer in the center of the parchment paper and fold the paper to cover the fish, sealing the edges to create a clamshell shape. Press the edges together firmly to ensure that steam and juices will not escape. Bake for approximately 15 minutes, or until the fish flakes easily with a fork. Cut a slit in the top of the parchment paper to release steam. Serve the fish atop the Coleslaw and garnish with cilantro.

COLESLAW

1 cup plain 2% Greek yogurt

¼ cup chopped fresh cilantro

1 clove garlic, minced

Juice of ½ lime

Sea salt and pepper to taste

2 cups red cabbage, shredded

In a large bowl, whisk together the yogurt, cilantro, garlic, lime juice and salt and pepper. Add the cabbage and toss to coat thoroughly.

Protein: 32.2 g | Carb: 15.5 g | Fat: 9.5 g | Fiber: 1.8 g

HEALTHY COBB SALAD (STARCHY CARB–FREE)

Serves 2

Olive oil cooking spray

4 strips low-fat nitrate-free turkey bacon

½ cup liquid egg whites

2 cups chopped lettuce

2 cups coleslaw mix

1 cooked boneless, skinless chicken breast (4–5 ounces), cubed

1 large tomato, chopped

¼ avocado, chopped

¼ cup chopped green onion

2 tablespoons crumbled goat-milk feta cheese

DRESSING

½ cup plain 0% Greek yogurt

1 teaspoon Dijon mustard

1 teaspoon fresh lemon juice

1 tablespoon chopped fresh chives

1 tablespoon dried parsley

2 teaspoons garlic powder

2 teaspoons onion powder
Sea salt and pepper to taste

Lightly grease a skillet with cooking spray and place over medium-high heat. Cook the turkey bacon until crispy, 2 to 3 minutes per side. Remove from the pan and blot on a paper towel; break into small pieces and set aside. Rinse the pan, then lightly grease with cooking spray and place over medium heat. Add the egg whites and scramble until the eggs are set; set aside.

Divide the lettuce and coleslaw mix evenly between two bowls. Arrange the chicken, tomato, avocado, green onion, turkey bacon, scrambled egg and feta in rows on top.

DRESSING: In a blender, combine the yogurt, Dijon mustard, lemon juice, chives, parsley, garlic powder, onion powder and salt and pepper. Blend thoroughly, adding extra lemon juice as needed to reach the desired consistency; drizzle over salad.

Protein: 24 g | Carb: 20.5 g | Fat: 12.1 g | Fiber: 2.7 g

PAN-SEARED SCALLOPS WITH CAULIFLOWER MASH AND SPINACH (STARCHY CARB–FREE)
Serves 2
8 sea scallops
Sea salt and pepper to taste
½ teaspoon unsalted butter
Microgreens or pea sprouts
Fresh lemon juice

CAULIFLOWER MASH
3 cups cauliflower florets
1 tablespoon coconut milk
½ teaspoon unsalted butter
Pinch each of sea salt and black or white pepper

SPINACH

½ teaspoon unsalted butter

1 clove garlic, minced

2 bunches fresh spinach, trimmed

CAULIFLOWER MASH: Steam the cauliflower until soft; transfer to the bowl of a food processor and purée until smooth. Transfer the cauliflower to a medium saucepan and stir in the coconut milk, butter and salt and pepper. Cover the pan and keep warm over low heat until needed.

SPINACH: In a large skillet, melt the butter over medium-high heat. Add the garlic and sauté for 1 minute. Add the spinach and cook until wilted, about 3 minutes; cover and set aside.

Pat the scallops dry and sprinkle with salt and pepper. In a medium skillet, melt the butter over medium-high heat; when the foam subsides, add the scallops to the pan and sear them on both sides until cooked through. To serve, spoon the Cauliflower Mash into the middle of each plate, add a nest of spinach, then top with the scallops. Garnish with microgreens or pea sprouts and a squeeze of lemon juice.

Protein: 24 g | Carb: 15.6 g | Fat: 14.8 g | Fiber: 4g

EGG PEPPER POCKETS WITH TURKEY BACON (STARCHY CARB–FREE)

Serves 2

2 red or yellow bell peppers

Olive oil cooking spray

4 eggs

2 tablespoons Mrs. Dash Original Blend

Garlic powder, to taste

4 strips low-fat nitrate-free turkey bacon

2 cups mixed greens

Fresh chives, to taste

Slice the peppers to make four 1½-inch-thick rings (in which the eggs will cook). Lightly grease a large skillet with cooking spray and place over medium heat. Place the pepper rings in the pan and crack an egg into each ring slowly, so that the pepper forms a seal. Cook for 3 to 4 minutes, and then flip them over to cook the other side. When the eggs are cooked to your preference, sprinkle with Mrs. Dash and garlic powder.

Meanwhile, in a separate skillet, cook the turkey bacon according to package directions. Serve the eggs on a bed of mixed greens, with a sprinkle of fresh chives and the turkey bacon on the side.

Protein: 23.3 g | Carb: 15.1 g | Fat: 14.1 g | Fiber: 2.5 g

TUNA POWER BOWL (STARCHY CARB–FREE)
Serves 2
3 cups mixed greens or kale

½ cup diced cucumber

½ cup halved cherry tomatoes

¼ cup chopped celery

¼ avocado, chopped

2 tablespoons chives

1 can light tuna, in water, broken into chunks

1 tablespoon extra-virgin olive oil

1 tablespoon rice wine vinegar

Juice of ½ lemon

1 teaspoon unpasteurized honey

1 teaspoon dried dill

½ teaspoon ground ginger

Layer the greens in the bottom of a salad bowl and top with the cucumber, cherry tomatoes, celery, avocado, chives and tuna. In a small bowl, whisk together the oil, rice wine vinegar, lemon juice, honey, dill and ginger; drizzle over salad.

Protein: 22.5 g | Carb: 16.9 g | Fat: 11.5 g | Fiber: 2.8 g

BETTA BRUSCHETTA CHICKEN (STARCHY CARB–FREE)
Serves 3
This meal can also be cooked on the grill.

3 boneless, skinless chicken breasts (4–6 ounces each)
Sea salt and pepper to taste
1 bunch baby spinach
4 small tomatoes, chopped
1 red, yellow or orange bell pepper, chopped
1 small red onion, chopped
3 cloves garlic, minced
Handful fresh basil, chopped
2 tablespoons extra-virgin olive oil
1 teaspoon balsamic vinegar
$\frac{1}{8}$ teaspoon sea salt

Preheat oven to 400°F. Season the chicken with salt and pepper and place on a parchment paper–lined baking sheet; bake for 20 to 25 minutes or until cooked through. Meanwhile, in a large bowl, combine the spinach, tomatoes, bell pepper, red onion, garlic, basil, oil, balsamic vinegar and salt. In a skillet over medium-low heat, sauté the vegetable mixture until warmed through. Spoon the bruschetta topping over the chicken breasts.

Protein: 27.6 g | Carb: 18 g | Fat: 11 g | Fiber: 2.3 g

SALMON PATTIES WITH SIMPLE TARTAR SAUCE (STARCHY CARB–FREE)

Serves 4

You can substitute tuna or any leftover fish for the salmon in this recipe.

16 ounces cooked wild salmon (about 4 fillets), coarsely flaked

2 whole eggs

½ red onion, finely chopped

4 tablespoons fresh chives, finely chopped (set aside 1 teaspoon for garnish)

4 cloves garlic, minced

3 tablespoons coconut flour

2 teaspoons Dijon mustard

Sea salt and pepper to taste

Coconut oil cooking spray

TARTAR SAUCE

¼ cup full-fat olive oil–based mayonnaise

2 tablespoons minced pickles of your choice

1 teaspoon lemon zest

½ teaspoon chopped fresh dill

¼ teaspoon sea salt

TARTAR SAUCE: In a small bowl, combine the mayonnaise, pickles, lemon zest, dill and salt; set aside in the refrigerator while you prepare the salmon patties.

In a medium bowl, combine the salmon, eggs, red onion, chives, garlic, coconut flour, Dijon mustard and salt and pepper. Form the mixture into four patties. Lightly grease a medium skillet with cooking spray and place over medium heat. When the pan is hot, cook the patties, browning well on one side before attempting to flip them over to brown the other side (or they may break). Serve them warm over salad greens or alongside any green vegetable or fermented vegetable like sauerkraut, and top with Tartar Sauce.

Protein: 28 g | Carb: 7 g | Fat: 14 g | Fiber: 5 g

OVEN-BAKED GOAT CHEESE, TOMATO AND SPINACH OMELET (STARCHY CARB–FREE)

Serves 1

Olive oil cooking spray

¼ cup chopped onion

½–1 cup chopped spinach

2 whole eggs and 1 egg white, whisked

6–8 grape tomatoes, halved

1 tablespoon soft goat cheese

Sea salt and pepper to taste

Dried basil to taste

Preheat oven to 400°F. Lightly grease a small ovenproof skillet with cooking spray and place over medium-high heat. Sauté the onion until translucent, 3 to 4 minutes. Add the spinach and cook until just wilted. Pour the eggs into the pan, add the grape tomatoes and dot with goat cheese. Sprinkle with salt, pepper and basil. Bake in the oven for 15 minutes. Serve immediately.

Protein: 21.4 g | Carb: 7.7 g | Fat: 12.7 g | Fiber: 2.6 g

CAST-IRON EGGY BAKE WITH RICOTTA (STARCHY CARB–FREE)

Serves 3

1 tablespoon extra-virgin olive oil

½ medium white onion, diced

1 clove garlic, minced

1 medium green or red bell pepper, chopped

4 cups diced tomatoes, or 2 cans (14 ounces each) diced tomatoes

2 tablespoons tomato paste

1 teaspoon chili powder

1 teaspoon cumin

1 teaspoon paprika

Sea salt and pepper

Pinch cayenne pepper

6 eggs

1 cup low-fat ricotta cheese

½ tablespoon chopped fresh parsley

In a deep, large skillet, heat the oil over medium heat. Add the chopped onion and sauté until it begins to soften, then add the garlic and continue to sauté for a few more minutes. Add the bell pepper and sauté for an additional 5 to 7 minutes, until tender-crisp. Add the tomatoes and tomato paste and stir to combine. Add the chili powder, cumin and paprika and stir to combine; simmer for 5 to 7 minutes, until the liquid begins to reduce. Add salt and pepper to taste, as well as the pinch of cayenne. Crack the eggs directly into the sauce, spacing them evenly in the pan. Cover and allow the eggs to cook for 10 to 12 minutes, or according to your preference. Dollop the ricotta over the tomato mixture and heat through. Remove from the heat, garnish with parsley and serve immediately.

Protein: 19.9 g | Carb: 12.2 g | Fat: 13 g | Fiber: 2.5 g

SASSY SOLE WITH ZUCCHINI AND OLIVES (STARCHY CARB–FREE)

Serves 1

1 sole fillet (4–5 ounces)

¼ teaspoon sea salt

¼ teaspoon pepper

1 cup halved cherry tomatoes

1 small zucchini, finely chopped

2 tablespoons capers, undrained

5 olives, sliced

1 teaspoon extra-virgin olive oil

Preheat oven to 425°F. Sprinkle both sides of the fish with salt and pepper and place on an 11- x 7-inch rimmed baking sheet lined with parchment paper. In a small bowl, combine the cherry tomatoes, zucchini, capers, olives and oil; spoon over fish. Bake for 22 minutes and serve immediately.

Protein: 29.3 g | Carb: 21.4 g | Fat: 18.4 g | Fiber: 3 g

ASIAN SIRLOIN STEAK (STARCHY CARB–FREE)
Serves 2

½ cup cooking sherry

¼ cup gluten-free tamari soy sauce

2 tablespoons honey

1 tablespoon sesame oil

2 tablespoons (heaping) minced ginger root

2 tablespoons minced garlic (3–5 cloves)

½ teaspoon red pepper flakes

2 grass-fed sirloin steaks (4–5 ounces each)

1 tablespoon sesame seeds, toasted

2 green onions, sliced

In a shallow dish, whisk together the sherry, soy sauce, honey, sesame oil, ginger, garlic and red pepper flakes. Add the steaks, turning to coat, and cover and refrigerate for 3 to 4 hours. Grill the steaks on high heat for 4 minutes per side (for medium-rare). Allow them to rest for 5 minutes before slicing and serving. Garnish with toasted sesame seeds and green onions. Serve with Cauliflower Mash (page 284) and a baby arugula salad (1 to 2 cups per person).

Protein: 34 g | Carb: 25.4 g | Fat: 15.1 g | Fiber: 2.1 g

ZUCCHINI PASTA AND TURKEY ROSÉ SAUCE (STARCHY CARB–FREE)

Serves 4

This recipe can be made with beef, bison, veal or chicken instead of turkey.

2 tablespoons unsalted butter or ghee

1 onion, finely diced

1 carrot, finely diced or grated

1 celery stalk, finely diced

6 cloves garlic, minced

¼ teaspoon dried basil

Sea salt and pepper to taste

½ pound ground turkey

1 can (28 ounces) organic Roma tomatoes (no salt added)

3 ounces (or ½ small can) tomato paste

½ cup low-fat canned coconut milk

6 medium zucchini

Coconut oil cooking spray

In a large skillet over medium-high heat, melt the butter or ghee. Sauté the onions, carrot and celery until softened. Add the garlic, basil, salt and pepper. Add the turkey and cook until browned. Add the tomatoes, tomato paste and coconut milk; bring to a boil. Turn down the heat to medium-low and simmer for 20 to 30 minutes. While the sauce is reducing, spiralize the zucchini. Lightly grease a separate skillet with cooking spray and place over high heat. Add the zucchini and sauté for 5 minutes. Check the sauce and add salt and pepper to taste. When the sauce reaches the desired thickness, remove from the heat. Plate the zucchini noodles, top with sauce and serve.

Protein: 22.5 g | Carb: 21.7 g | Fat: 7.2 g | Fiber: 6.1 g

FLANK STEAK WITH ROMESCO SAUCE AND CAULIFLOWER MASH (STARCHY CARB–FREE)

Serves 3–4

This recipe is also delicious made with boneless, skinless chicken breasts instead of steak.

1 tablespoon unsalted butter

3 grass-fed flank steaks (4–5 ounces each)

Sea salt and pepper to taste

1 bundle asparagus, trimmed

Cauliflower Mash (page 284)

ROMESCO SAUCE

1 red bell pepper, cut in half and seeded

1 cup cherry tomatoes

$\frac{1}{4}$ cup raw whole almonds

4 cloves garlic, peeled

1 tablespoon red wine vinegar

2 teaspoons extra-virgin olive oil

$\frac{1}{4}$ teaspoon smoked paprika

$\frac{1}{4}$ teaspoon sea salt

$\frac{1}{8}$ teaspoon cayenne pepper

ROMESCO SAUCE: Heat the broiler. Place the bell pepper halves cut side down on a baking sheet lined with parchment paper and broil 4 inches from the heat until charred, about 20 minutes. Transfer to a bowl, cover with plastic wrap, and allow to steam until cool enough to handle. Peel off the skin and set the peppers aside. Turn the oven temperature to 375°F. Place the cherry tomatoes, almonds and garlic cloves on a baking sheet lined with parchment paper; bake for 10 minutes. Remove the almonds and return the baking sheet to the oven for another 15 minutes. In the bowl of a food processor, combine the roasted red pepper halves, cherry tomatoes, almonds, garlic, red wine vinegar, oil, paprika, salt and cayenne; purée until desired consistency is reached, then set aside.

In a large skillet, melt the butter over medium-high heat. Sprinkle both sides of the steaks with salt and pepper and, when the pan is very hot, add the steaks. Sear for about 5 minutes per side, or until desired doneness. Transfer to a cutting board and tent with foil. To the same skillet over medium heat, add the asparagus and sprinkle with a bit of salt; sauté for 5 to 7 minutes, or until tender-crisp. Thinly slice the steak against the grain. Plate the Cauliflower Mash and asparagus stalks as a bed for the steak, then top with Romesco Sauce.

Protein: 29.2 g | Carb:13.6 g | Fat: 9.9 g | Fiber: 5.9 g

PAELLA AND CAULIFLOWER RICE (STARCHY CARB–FREE)
Serves 4

4 cups low-sodium chicken or vegetable stock

3–4 tablespoons extra-virgin olive oil

3 onions, chopped

1½ green bell peppers, chopped

1½ red bell peppers, chopped

6 cloves garlic, minced

1 can (28 ounces) diced organic tomatoes, drained

4 bay leaves

2–3 tablespoons no-salt Cajun seasoning

Smoked paprika, celery salt, salt, pepper and red pepper flakes to taste

1½ heads cauliflower, "riced" using a food processor

1 pound shrimp (approximately 4 per serving), peeled and deveined

Fresh parsley, chopped

2 lemons, cut into wedges

In a medium saucepan over medium-high heat, bring the chicken stock to a simmer. In a large skillet, heat the oil over medium heat. Sauté the onions, bell peppers and garlic until softened. Add the tomatoes, bay leaves, Cajun seasoning, and other spices to taste. Then stir in the cauliflower and hot stock. Add the shrimp and cook for 3 minutes or until pink, stirring occasionally. Serve topped with parsley and a generous amount of juice from the lemon wedges.

Protein: 27.3 g | Carb: 28.1 g | Fat: 10.3 g | Fiber: 9.6 g

Starchy Carb Meal Options (Meal 4)

TURMERIC AND CANNELLINI BEAN STEW (STARCHY CARB MEAL)
Serves 4

3 tablespoons coconut oil
1 cup diced white onions
1 cup diced carrots
3 cloves garlic, minced
1 jalapeno pepper, minced
1 can (28 ounces) diced organic tomatoes
1 cup canned organic cannellini beans, rinsed and drained
1 can (14 ounces) low-sodium vegetable stock
3 tablespoons ground turmeric
2 teaspoons ground cumin
1 teaspoon chili powder
$\frac{1}{4}$ teaspoon sea salt
3 boneless, skinless chicken breasts (4–6 ounces each), cubed
1½ heads cauliflower, cut up into florets
1 cup cooked quinoa, hot

In a large saucepan, heat the coconut oil over medium-high heat. Add the onions, carrots, garlic and jalapeno sauté for 5 minutes or until softened. Stir in the tomatoes, beans, vegetable stock, turmeric, cumin, chili powder and salt; bring to a boil. Reduce the heat. Add the chicken; cover and simmer for 15 to 20 minutes. Add the cauliflower during the last 10 minutes of cooking time. Serve with quinoa.

Protein: 29.1 g | Carb: 35.2 g | Fat: 13.8 g | Fiber: 8.1 g

STUFFED PEPPERS (STARCHY CARB MEAL)
Serves 6
Coconut oil cooking spray
1 tablespoon coconut oil
1 large onion, diced
4 cloves garlic, minced
1 pound ground turkey
1 teaspoon dried oregano
½ teaspoon turmeric
½ teaspoon sea salt
Pepper to taste
1 cup cooked quinoa
2 large zucchini, diced
3 tablespoons tomato paste
6 large bell peppers (any color—though green is lowest-carb option),
    tops cut off and seeded
½ cup goat-milk mozzarella, grated
Fresh parsley, chopped

Preheat oven to 350°F. Lightly grease a baking dish (large enough to hold 6 stuffed peppers) with cooking spray and set aside. Bring a large pot of water to a boil. Meanwhile, in a large skillet, heat the coconut oil over medium heat. Add the onion and garlic and sauté for 3 to 4 minutes, until softened. Add the turkey, oregano, turmeric, salt and pepper and cook until the turkey is browned. As the turkey finishes cooking, add the quinoa and zucchini. Continue cooking until the zucchini is tender-crisp. Remove the pan from the heat, drain the juices and stir in the tomato paste.

Place the bell peppers upright in the baking dish and spoon the turkey mixture into each pepper. Bake for 25 minutes. Top with the cheese for the last few minutes of cooking time. Serve warm, sprinkled with chopped parsley.

Protein: 29.6 g | Carb: 18.1 g | Fat: 12.5 g | Fiber: 4.3 g

CHICKEN AND LENTIL CHARD SOUP (STARCHY CARB MEAL)
Serves 4

4 tablespoons extra-virgin olive oil

1 medium white onion, diced

1 carrot, diced

4 cloves garlic, minced

2 teaspoons ground cumin

1 teaspoon curry powder

½ teaspoon dried thyme

1 can (28 ounces) diced organic tomatoes, drained

1 cup canned organic green or brown lentils, rinsed and drained

4 cups low-sodium vegetable stock

2 cups water

1 teaspoon sea salt (or more, to taste)

Pinch red pepper flakes

Freshly ground black pepper

2 cups Swiss chard, chopped

4 cooked boneless, skinless chicken breasts (4–5 ounces each), diced

Juice of ½ to 1 lemon

In a large pot or Dutch oven, heat the oil over medium heat. Add the onion and carrot and cook until the onion is translucent. Add the garlic, cumin, curry powder and thyme. Add the tomatoes and cook for a few more minutes, stirring often. Add the lentils, stock, water, salt and red pepper flakes. Season generously with freshly ground black pepper. Raise the heat and bring the mixture to a boil, then partially cover the pot and reduce the heat to maintain a gentle simmer. Cook for 30 minutes. Transfer 2 cups of the soup to a blender. Protecting your hand from the heat, purée the soup until smooth (to add thickness). Pour the puréed soup back into the pot and add the chard and cooked chicken. Remove the pot from the heat and stir in the lemon juice. Season with more salt and pepper, if necessary.

Protein: 34.6 g | Carb: 24.7 g | Fat: 14.5 g | Fiber: 8.2 g

TUSCAN ONE-POT HALIBUT (STARCHY CARB MEAL)
Serves 5

2 tablespoons extra-virgin olive oil
1 cup sliced button mushrooms
½ yellow onion, diced
2 cloves garlic, minced
2 Atlantic halibut fillets (10–12 ounces each)
¼ teaspoon dried oregano
¼ teaspoon dried thyme
¼ teaspoon sea salt
¼ teaspoon pepper
¼ teaspoon red pepper flakes (optional)
1 can (28 ounces) diced organic tomatoes
¾ cup cannellini beans, rinsed and drained
¼ cup sliced sun-dried tomatoes
1 teaspoon coconut sugar
Sea salt and pepper
2 to 3 cups cooked quinoa, hot
Parsley, chopped

In a large, deep skillet, heat the oil over high heat. Add the mushrooms and sauté until the liquid has evaporated and they are browned. Add the onion and garlic and lower the heat to medium. Add the fish; when it is partly cooked, add the oregano, thyme, salt, pepper and red pepper flakes (if using). Then add the canned tomatoes, beans and sun-dried tomatoes. Add the coconut sugar (to balance acids) and salt and pepper to taste. Serve with ¼ to ½ cup of cooked quinoa per serving, and garnish with parsley.

Protein: 36.2 g | Carb: 39.6 g | Fat: 9.5 g | Fiber: 5.2 g

SQUASH NEST SPICY GARLIC SHRIMP (STARCHY-CARB MEAL)
Serves 4

Olive oil cooking spray
2 spaghetti squash, halved lengthwise and seeded
Sea salt and pepper to taste
2 tablespoons extra-virgin olive oil
½ cup diced yellow onion
4 large cloves garlic, minced
1 can (28 ounces) crushed organic tomatoes
½ teaspoon red pepper flakes
1 teaspoon sea salt
1 teaspoon dried basil
1 teaspoon dried oregano
½ teaspoon dried parsley
½ cup low-sodium chicken stock
1 cup plain 0% or 2% Greek yogurt, at room temperature
1 pound shrimp, peeled and deveined
2 tablespoons pumpkin seeds

Preheat oven to 375°F. Line a baking sheet with foil and lightly grease with cooking spray. Season the squash with salt and pepper and place cut side down on the baking sheet. Bake for 40 minutes, or until the squash is tender.

While the squash is baking, prepare the shrimp. In a large skillet, heat the oil over medium heat. Add the onion and cook for about 3 minutes, until translucent. Add the garlic and cook for another minute. Add the tomatoes, red pepper flakes, salt, basil, oregano and parsley; stir. Simmer over medium-low heat for about 5 minutes. Stir in the chicken stock, then remove from the heat. Add the yogurt and stir until it is incorporated and the sauce is smooth. Stir in the shrimp. Turn the heat back up to medium and simmer until the shrimp is cooked, about 5 minutes. Serve the shrimp inside the prepared spaghetti squash nests, or remove the squash flesh onto a plate and top with spicy shrimp. Sprinkle with pumpkin seeds.

Protein: 31.5 g | Carb: 27 g | Fat: 11 g | Fiber: 5.1 g

SLOW COOKER BEEF STEW (STARCHY CARB MEAL)
Serves 6
4 cups low-sodium beef stock

1 can (15 ounces) diced organic tomatoes

5–6 small red potatoes, unpeeled and quartered

2 cups baby carrots

1 celery stalk, chopped

3 tablespoons tomato paste

3 teaspoons Italian seasoning

½ cup flour

Sea salt and pepper

1½ pounds beef stew meat

1½ tablespoons olive oil, divided

1 white or yellow onion, chopped

In a slow cooker, combine the beef stock, tomatoes, potatoes, carrots, celery, tomato paste and Italian seasoning. In a bowl, combine the flour with salt and pepper to taste. Add the beef to the flour mixture and toss to coat. In a skillet, heat 1 tablespoon of the oil over medium heat and brown the beef chunks on all sides, then add them to the slow cooker. In a separate skillet, heat the remaining ½ tablespoon of oil and sauté the onion until it is translucent; transfer it to the slow cooker. Cover and cook on Low for 6 to 8 hours. Stir, add salt and pepper to taste and serve.

Protein: 43 g | Carb: 35.9 g | Fat: 9.8 g | Fiber: 5.3 g

ONE-POT PAPRIKA CHICKEN (STARCHY CARB MEAL)

Serves 4

4 tablespoons smoked paprika

Sea salt and pepper to taste

4 boneless, skinless chicken breasts (4–5 ounces each)

2 tablespoons extra-virgin olive oil

1 medium onion, finely chopped

2 tablespoons minced garlic

2 cups sliced button mushrooms

4 small red potatoes, unpeeled and chopped into small chunks

3 carrots, sliced

2 tablespoons coconut, almond or other gluten-free flour

1/4 cup dry white wine

1/2 cup low-sodium chicken stock

1 1/2 tablespoons chopped fresh thyme

2 cups cooked quinoa, hot

In a resealable plastic bag, combine the paprika with salt and pepper. Add the chicken breasts, one at a time, and shake to coat thoroughly in the spice mixture, adding more spices if needed to coat all the pieces. In a large skillet, heat the oil over medium-high heat. Cook the chicken for 2 minutes on each side, until browned. Transfer to a plate. In the same pan, sauté the onion and garlic for 2 minutes, then add the mushrooms and continue to sauté, stirring, for another 2 minutes. Add the potatoes and carrots. Sprinkle with salt and pepper and sauté for about 5 minutes. In a small bowl, whisk the flour together with the wine. Pour slowly over the vegetables, stirring, then add the chicken stock and bring to a boil. Return the chicken to the pan, cover, and reduce the heat to medium, simmering until the chicken and vegetables are cooked, about 30 minutes. Sprinkle with fresh thyme and serve on a bed of 1/2 cup quinoa.

Protein: 32 g | Carb: 34 g | Fat: 11.3 g | Fiber: 4.5 g

MUSHROOM CHICKEN QUINOA RISOTTO (STARCHY CARB MEAL)

Serves 3

2 tablespoons extra-virgin olive oil

1 pound button mushrooms, sliced

3 shallots, diced

3 cloves garlic, minced

2 tablespoons white wine vinegar

1 cup quinoa, rinsed

1 cup water

1 cup low-sodium chicken or vegetable stock

Coconut oil cooking spray

3 boneless, skinless chicken breasts (4–5 ounces each)

2 sprigs fresh tarragon

In a large skillet, heat the oil over high heat. Add the mushrooms and cook for about 5 to 10 minutes, or until the liquid has evaporated and the mushrooms are browned. Add the shallots and garlic and sauté until the onion is translucent. Add the white wine vinegar and cook for 2 minutes. Add the quinoa, water and chicken stock; cover and cook for 5 to 7 minutes, until the quinoa is done. Meanwhile, in a medium skillet lightly greased with cooking spray, cook the chicken breasts on both sides until they are done. Fluff the quinoa with a fork, top with the chicken and garnish with tarragon.

Protein: 34 g | Carb: 20.7 g | Fat: 13 g | Fiber: 3.2 g

COCONUT CURRY BUTTERNUT CHICKEN SOUP (STARCHY CARB MEAL)

Serves 4

1 tablespoon extra-virgin olive oil

1 medium white onion, diced

3 celery stalks, diced

2 tablespoons curry powder

1 teaspoon turmeric

1 teaspoon cumin

1 teaspoon coriander

1 large butternut squash (about 3 pounds), cubed

¼ cup water

½ cup light coconut milk (canned)

2 teaspoons sea salt

2 tablespoons freshly squeezed lemon juice

3 boneless, skinless chicken breasts (4–5 ounces each), cubed

Sea salt and pepper to taste

Coconut oil cooking spray

¾ cup plain 2% Greek yogurt

¼ cup chopped fresh cilantro

In a soup pot, heat the oil over high heat and sauté the onion until translucent, about 5 minutes. Add the celery, curry powder, turmeric, cumin and coriander; sauté for 5 minutes. Add the squash and sauté for about 10 to 12 minutes, until softened. Add the water to the pot, cover, and cook until the vegetables are very tender, stirring occasionally (add more water if needed). Remove from the heat and transfer the vegetables to the bowl of a food processor; process until smooth. (Alternatively, you can blend the vegetables in the pot with a hand blender. Be careful; it will be very hot.) Return the puréed vegetables to the pot over medium heat and add the coconut milk and 2 teaspoons of salt; whisk until well blended. Heat until the soup is warm. Stir in the lemon juice.

While the soup is heating, season the chicken cubes with salt, pepper and additional curry powder. Cook the chicken in a skillet lightly greased with cooking spray. When ready to serve, spoon the soup into bowls, topping each with the cooked chicken, yogurt and cilantro.

Protein: 26.6 g | Carb: 30 g | Fat: 13.1 g | Fiber: 3.9 g

FAKE-OUT TAKEOUT BEEF AND BROCCOLI (STARCHY CARB MEAL)

Serves 5

1 cup low-sodium beef consommé or stock

½ cup low-sodium, gluten-free tamari soy sauce

2 tablespoons honey

1 tablespoon sesame oil

3 cloves garlic, minced

25–30 ounces boneless beef chuck roast, sliced into thin strips (about
     5–6 ounces per person)

2 tablespoons coconut flour

3 cups frozen or fresh broccoli florets

2 cups cooked white or brown basmati rice, hot

In a slow cooker, whisk together the beef consommé, soy sauce, honey, sesame oil and garlic. Add the beef and toss to coat. Cook on low for 6 hours. In a small bowl, whisk together the coconut flour and ½ cup of the cooking liquid; stir it into the slow cooker, mixing well. Cook on Low for an additional 30 minutes to thicken the sauce. In the last 10 minutes of cooking, add the broccoli. Serve the beef hot over rice.

Protein: 37.3 g | Carb: 44.3 g | Fat: 14 g | Fiber: 3 g

Smoothies

Unless otherwise stated, the smoothie-making method is the same for all the recipes in this section. Start by blending all the listed ingredients *except* your protein supplement. Then add the powder and briefly blend again. This will prevent damage to the protein, which could happen with over-blending.

I have listed a protein powder flavor for each recipe, but I purposely did not specify the type. It's up to you to choose your preference from the list of Foods to Enjoy. Your options include whey, hemp, rice, pea or any other vegan protein base, except soy.

Also, try not to think of ground flax or chia as suitable replacements for the fiber supplement. Most supplements provide double the amount of fiber found in 2 tablespoons of seeds. I prefer that you save the seeds for sprinkling on your meals. Doing so will provide you with regular doses of fiber throughout the day—a definite benefit, since it makes you feel full and causes the release of your fat-burning friend adiponectin.

A final note regarding the nutrition content of the fruit-free smoothie recipes: These are slightly higher in protein and fat to make up for the lower amount of carbohydrate in the mix. Remember, skipping fruit or other carbs at breakfast helps to keep you in the ketogenic (fat-burning) state that occurs overnight and which will last until your first carb-containing meal of the day. If you feel your results are slowing down or if you hit a weight-loss plateau, you may want to kick in the carb-free breakfast as a means of tricking your metabolism.

CHOCO BANANA-RAMA SMOOTHIE

½ frozen banana

1 cup unsweetened almond milk

1 tablespoon organic almond butter

1 tablespoon raw cacao powder

Cinnamon to taste

1 serving fiber supplement

1 cup ice or water

1 serving chocolate protein powder

Protein: 29.4 g | Carb: 17.4 g | Fat: 14.5 g | Fiber: 11.6 g

MATCHA MADNESS SMOOTHIE

¼ cup frozen strawberries

1 cup unsweetened almond or cashew milk

2 tablespoons hemp seeds

1 teaspoon matcha (green tea powder)

1 teaspoon spirulina

1 serving fiber supplement

1 cup ice or water

1 serving vanilla protein powder

Protein: 33 g | Carb: 23.2 g | Fat: 11.6 g | Fiber: 8 g

APPLE PIE SMOOTHIE

Tip: This smoothie may also be served warm.

1 cup Royal Gala apple slices

1–2 cups cool or warmed unsweetened almond milk

1 tablespoon raw walnut butter or 6 walnut halves

1 teaspoon cinnamon

1 serving fiber supplement

1 serving vanilla protein powder

Protein: 28.3 g | Carb: 27 g | Fat: 12.3 g | Fiber: 10.5 g

PEACH-COLADA SMOOTHIE

½ cup spinach

1 small peach, pitted and sliced

1 teaspoon unsweetened shredded coconut

½ cup unsweetened coconut milk (from a carton)

2 tablespoons hemp seeds

1 serving fiber supplement

Ice or water as needed

1 serving vanilla protein powder

Protein: 34.7 g | Carb: 24 g | Fat: 12.6 g | Fiber: 11 g

BANANA "CREAM PIE" SMOOTHIE

½ frozen or fresh banana

1 cup unsweetened vanilla almond milk

1 tablespoon hemp seeds

1 teaspoon vanilla extract

½ teaspoon cinnamon

¼ teaspoon nutmeg

1 serving fiber supplement

1 heaping cup ice (adjust to fit your desired consistency)

1 serving vanilla protein powder

Protein: 30.1 g | Carb: 19 g | Fat: 6.8 g | Fiber: 9.8 g

COCOA HEMP CINNA-BLISS SMOOTHIE (FRUIT-FREE)

⅔ cup unsweetened chocolate almond milk

2 tablespoons hemp seeds

2 tablespoons raw cacao powder

1 tablespoon cinnamon

1 serving fiber supplement

Ice cubes and water to taste

1 serving chocolate protein powder

Protein: 34.7 g | Carb: 18 g | Fat: 12.2 g | Fiber: 9 g

PUMPKIN PIE SMOOTHIE (FRUIT-FREE)

½ cup unsweetened pumpkin purée

½ cup unsweetened vanilla almond milk

½ cup plain 2% Greek yogurt

2 tablespoons hemp seeds

1 teaspoon vanilla extract

1 teaspoon nutmeg

1 teaspoon cinnamon

1 serving fiber supplement

¼ cup ice

1 serving vanilla protein powder

Protein: 31.6 g | Carb: 26.5 g | Fat: 13.4 g | Fiber: 8 g

GINGERBREAD SMOOTHIE

½ frozen banana

1 cup unsweetened vanilla almond milk

2 tablespoons hemp seeds

1 teaspoon vanilla extract

½ teaspoon cinnamon

½ teaspoon ground ginger

¼ teaspoon nutmeg

⅛ teaspoon ground cloves

1 serving fiber supplement

1 cup ice

1 serving vanilla protein powder

Protein: 26.7 g | Carb: 26 g | Fat: 10.9 g | Fiber: 9.8 g

PEAR AND BASIL SMOOTHIE

1 small pear (Asian pears are the highest-fiber option)

Handful basil

12 raw cashews

1 cup unsweetened almond milk

1 serving fiber supplement

2 ice cubes

1 serving vanilla protein powder

Protein: 31.7 g | Carb: 31.6 g | Fat: 15 g | Fiber: 13.4 g

CHOCOLATE CHERRY DELIGHT

½ cup frozen pitted cherries

Small bunch baby kale

¼ cup unsweetened coconut milk (from a carton)

1 tablespoon hemp seeds

1 serving fiber supplement

1 serving chocolate protein powder

Protein: 31 g | Carb: 23 g | Fat: 8.3 g | Fiber: 8 g

STRAWBERRY GINGER TURMARIKA SMOOTHIE

¼ cup strawberries

1 cup unsweetened vanilla almond milk

2 tablespoons hemp seeds

1 teaspoon turmeric

½ teaspoon cinnamon

½ teaspoon ground ginger (or you can use sliced ginger root)

1 serving fiber supplement

1 serving vanilla protein powder

Protein: 32.7 g | Carb: 23.2 g | Fat: 11.2 g | Fiber: 8 g

GREEN LEAP AVOCADO SMOOTHIE (FRUIT-FREE)

¼ avocado

½ cup fresh baby spinach or kale

¼ cup fresh mint

¼ cup organic light coconut milk (from a carton)

2 tablespoons unsalted pistachio nuts

2 tablespoons hemp seeds

1 vanilla bean (or ½ teaspoon vanilla extract)

1 serving fiber supplement

½ cup water

Ice cubes (as many as you like)

1 serving vanilla protein powder

Protein: 34.1 g | Carb: 21.2 g | Fat: 15.3 g | Fiber: 8 g

DR. TURNER'S FAVORITE BLUEBERRY SPINACH SMOOTHIE

½ cup frozen blueberries

½–1 cup organic baby spinach

1 cup water or low-carb milk (almond or cashew)

2 tablespoons hemp seeds

½–1 teaspoon cinnamon

1 serving fiber supplement

1 serving vanilla protein powder

Protein: 35.7 g | Carb: 30 g | Fat: 11.1 g | Fiber: 9.8 g

CAFÉ AU LAIT (FRUIT-FREE)

1–2 tablespoons organic instant coffee or Swiss water–processed decaf
   instant coffee, or about ½ cup brewed coffee

1 tablespoon unsweetened cacao nibs

1 cup unsweetened almond milk (less if using brewed coffee)

1 tablespoon almond or hazelnut butter (or 2 tablespoons hemp seeds)

Cinnamon to taste

1 serving fiber supplement

1 serving chocolate or vanilla protein powder

Protein: 34 g | Carb: 16 g | Fat: 16.5 g | Fiber: 9.5 g

MINT CHOCOLATE CHIP SMOOTHIE (FRUIT-FREE)

½ small avocado (or ¼ regular-sized one)

1 cup unsweetened vanilla almond milk

¼ cup peppermint herbal tea

1 teaspoon cacao powder or 1 tablespoon unsweetened cacao nibs

3–5 drops peppermint oil

1 serving fiber supplement

1 serving chocolate protein powder

Protein: 33 g | Carb: 16 g | Fat: 12.5 g | Fiber: 9 g

DARK CHOCOLATE SALTY CRUNCH SMOOTHIE (FRUIT-FREE)

1 tablespoon organic almond butter

1 tablespoon cacao nibs

1 cup unsweetened chocolate almond milk

Pinch sea salt

1 serving fiber supplement

1 serving chocolate protein powder

Protein: 37 g | Carb: 20 g | Fat: 16.5 g | Fiber: 9 g

GREENA-COLADA (FRUIT-FREE)

Handful of kale or spinach

1 tablespoon unsweetened shredded coconut

½ cup unsweetened vanilla almond milk

Dash each nutmeg and cinnamon

1 tablespoon hemp seeds

1 serving fiber supplement

1 serving vanilla protein powder

Protein: 32 g | Carb: 15.5 g | Fat: 16.5 g | Fiber: 8 g

SNICKERDOODLE CASHEW SMOOTHIE (FRUIT-FREE)

1 tablespoon cashew butter

1 cup unsweetened vanilla almond or coconut milk

1 tablespoon hemp seeds

1 teaspoon cinnamon

1 teaspoon vanilla extract

1 serving fiber supplement

1 serving vanilla protein powder

Protein: 37 g | Carb: 16 g | Fat: 14.7 g | Fiber: 9 g

CARROT CAKE SMOOTHIE (FRUIT-FREE)

½ cup shredded carrots

1 tablespoon unsweetened shredded coconut

¼ cup unsweetened almond milk

2 tablespoons walnuts

2 teaspoons coconut oil

1 teaspoon cinnamon

Nutmeg to taste

1 serving fiber supplement

Water as needed

1 serving vanilla protein powder

Protein: 33.2 g | Carb: 17.2 g | Fat: 19.3 g | Fiber: 8 g

THE HORMONE BOOST
SUCCESS TRACKER

Your time is limited; don't waste it living someone else's life. Don't be trapped by dogma, which is living the result of other people's thinking. Don't let the noise of other opinions drown your own inner voice. And most important, have the courage to follow your heart and intuition; they somehow already know what you truly want to become. Everything else is secondary.

STEVE JOBS,
co-founder of Apple Inc.

Why Use This—or Any—Tracker?

Did you know that keeping a food diary can double your success in weight loss? Well, it's true, according to a study from the Kaiser Permanente Center for Health Research. The findings, from one of the largest and longest-running weight-loss maintenance trials ever conducted at the time, were published in the August 2008 issue of the *American Journal of Preventive Medicine*. Those who kept daily food records lost twice as much weight as those who kept no records. It seems that the simple act of writing down what we eat (i.e., being aware of what and how much we eat), encourages us to consume less.

Another group of researchers, from the Fred Hutchinson Cancer Research Center, identified some simple changes that go a long way toward helping women in particular achieve weight loss. If you want to lose weight, you should faithfully keep a food journal, avoid skipping meals and stay away from eating in restaurants—especially at lunch. These results appeared in the *Journal of the Academy of Nutrition and Dietetics* (2012) and noted that the specific aim of the study was to identify behaviors that support the global goal of calorie reduction. Specifically, they found that:

- Women who kept food journals consistently lost about six pounds *more* than those who did not.
- Women who reported skipping meals lost almost eight *fewer* pounds than women who did not.
- Women who ate out for lunch at least weekly lost on average five *fewer* pounds than those who ate out less frequently (eating out often, regardless of the meal, was associated with less weight loss, but the strongest association was observed with lunch).

At the study's end, the group's number one piece of advice for weight loss was to keep a food journal to meet nutritional goals. And once you take up this advice, don't stop anytime soon, because tracking helps both your short- and long-term outcomes. Researchers from the Miriam Hospital published results in the *American Journal of Preventive Medicine* (January 2014) from one of the first studies of its kind; they followed weight-loss maintenance for individuals over a 10-year period. Their results showed that long-term weight-loss maintenance is possible, *if* we stick to key health behaviors like recording our diet. Higher success was also related to consistent physical activity, self-weighing and adequate eating (rather than skipping meals or overeating).

I recommend weighing yourself and taking your abdomen circumference at the belly button a minimum of once a week, but you should track your general sense of wellness, your food intake and your workouts daily. Losing weight doesn't mean much, in my mind, if you experience fatigue, pain, digestive problems, mood swings or sleep problems on the diet or regimen you've chosen. These are the things I want you to score daily.

Why focus on all these other issues? Because losing weight is about more than simply ticking off pounds: it's also about behaviors and overall health. Becoming more aware of how your behaviors affect your goals and general sense of well-being will provide added support to your efforts. Self-tracking, for example, gives you immediate feedback on how your choices accelerate or hinder your progress. You can break your larger goals into smaller, more manageable daily targets and tweak weekly if needed. This can make dieting almost like a strategy game—and help you avoid the pain of regret or guilt! It also lets you be more flexible about your eating and exercise habits, which I believe is always a much more effective way to approach your new lifestyle.

Self-tracking also lets you put minor mistakes into perspective and take action to correct those mistakes. The act of recording your behaviors will generally help you eat to optimize the fat-loss six and exercise the right way, which will make you lose weight. You don't have to be obsessive, but you do need to be honest about serving sizes, toppings and how the food is prepared. Read labels! Be consistent; carry your Hormone Boost Tracker (in this book, or purchase a smaller one from my website) with you, or use a diet-tracking app on your smartphone like MyFitnessPal. Just be sure to change your profile settings to match the Hormone Boost guidelines for protein, carb, fat and fiber intake.

Even scribbling down what you eat on a Post-it note, sending yourself emails tallying each meal, or sending yourself a text message can suffice. You need to write down what you eat so you can reflect on it and see what works and what doesn't. I hear patients say almost daily that they can't lose weight. So it's important to give yourself the right tools and support to accomplish your goals. Numerous studies show that food journaling in conjunction with a weight-management program or group works best. The first study I mentioned had people check in with a group once a week in addition to keeping a food log. Why not form your own Hormone Boost group?

Comedian Jerry Seinfeld once revealed the secret he used to become a better comic. Every day that he wrote new material, he would make a satisfying red X on the calendar. After a while, the chain of X's was something he felt compelled to continue. Every day that you make it to the gym (or do any other activity that you're trying to make a habit), make a large red X on your calendar to hold yourself accountable and stay motivated. I have to say, I prefer to track my workouts like this rather than in the same place as my nutrition habits, because seeing the red X's on a calendar gives me immediate gratification and the motivation to continue.

Getting a boost requires you to be committed, organized and motivated. The Hormone Boost Tracker will help you in all three of these areas. Now let's review the things I want you to record.

Food and Drink Habits

Upon starting the plan, you will record *everything* that you eat and drink daily. Record eating times and food amounts. Note your intermittent fasting and cheat days. You also need to track your water intake. Not sure how much water you should be drinking? Calculate your required daily intake with this formula:

[Your weight] x 0.55 = number of ounces to drink daily
Number of ounces to drink daily/8 = number of cups you need daily

So, for a person who weighs 150 pounds, this is how it works:

150 x 0.55 = 82.5 ounces
82.5 ounces/8 = 10.31 cups per day (round up to 11)

Health Markers

We're going to work with a star system when it comes to your health markers. The goal is five-star days for sleep, energy, mood and your digestion that are also free (0-rated) of pain, hunger and cravings! Here's how to score:

Cravings: 0 if you have no cravings; 5 if you have a lot

Hunger: 0 if you have no feelings of excessive hunger; 5 if you have a lot

Pain: 0 if you have no pain; 5 if you have a lot

Sleep: 5 is excellent; 0 is insomnia (also note the hours slept)

Digestion: 5 if you are free of bloating or other issues; 0 means loose stools, constipation or discomfort with bloating or indigestion

Mood: 5 is happy; 0 is down, unmotivated, anxious or depressed

Energy: 5 is high energy; 0 is you crawling into bed at midday for a long nap

Weight and Abdominal (Belly Button) Measurement

I recommend that you weigh yourself at the beginning of each week only, though I know some people like to step on the scale daily during the program. Your weight is by no means the be-all, end-all measurement of your success during this process; how you feel daily and where you carry those few extra pounds are equally important. Here's a simple calculation to use to find your optimal waist size: divide your height in inches by half. That's your target number. For example, I am 62.5 inches tall; therefore, my optimal waist circumference is less than 31.25 inches.

Exercise Habits

Write down all of the exercise you do daily, including the type of activity, how long your session was, and its intensity. Identify whether it was cardio, yoga or strength training. If it was strength training, record details such as which workout you completed.

Stress Reduction

Take 10 minutes per day as *you* time. Meditate, visualize, write down your goals, focus on the positive, write in your gratitude journal—or just simply breathe. Arguably, this could be the most important thing you do each day. Or write a positive word in this space every day, so that you can change your negative self-talk. We can be, after all, our worst critics—or our best mentors.

The Hormone Boost Daily Success Tracker

*Weight*_____ *Waist:* _____ *[Repeat Weekly]*

Date: _____

Hours Slept: _____

Cravings: [None]   0 1 2 3 4 5 [A lot]
Hunger: [None]   0 1 2 3 4 5 [A lot]
Pain: [No Pain]   0 1 2 3 4 5 [A lot of pain]
Sleep: [Poor]   0 1 2 3 4 5 [Great]
Digestion: [Poor]   0 1 2 3 4 5 [Great]
Mood: [Poor]   0 1 2 3 4 5 [Great]
Energy: [Poor]   0 1 2 3 4 5 [Great]

Meal 1: Time _____

Meal 2: Time _____

Meal 3: Time _____

Meal 4: Time _____

Water: Cups
1 2 3 4 5 6 7 8 9 10 11 12 13 14

Supplements
Yes   No

Exercise   Strength   Cardio   Yoga
Notes:

Stress Reduction or Positive Word of Day:

RESOURCES

If you want to lift yourself up, lift up someone else.

BOOKER T. WASHINGTON,
African-American educator, author and presidential advisor

Canadian Compounding Pharmacy
   The AIM Clinic Pharmacy: www.aimclinicpharmacy.com
   Haber's Pharmacy: www.haberspharmacy.com
   Kripp's Pharmacy: www.krippspharmacy.com
   Smith's Pharmacy: www.smithspharmacy.com
   York Downs Pharmacy: www.yorkdownsrx.com

Infrared Sauna
   SaunaRay Far Infrared Saunas: www.saunaray.com

Body-Fat/Composition Analyzer
   Tanita home body-fat analyzer: www.tanita.com

Natural Skin Care and Makeup
   Naturopathica Environmental Defense Mask: www.naturopathica.com
   Korres lip balms and body products: www.korres.com
   Caudalie (toxin-free skin care): www.caudalie.com
   Juice Beauty (toxin-free skin care): www.juicebeauty.com
   John Masters Organics (toxin-free skin and hair care):
      www.johnmasters.com
   Burt's Bees natural skin care: www.burtsbees.com
   Alba Botanica Sugar Cane Body Polish and Kukui Nut Hawaiian Body
      Oil: www.albabotanica.com
      (Unlike the two products listed here, not all Alba products are free of
      harmful methylparabens and propylparabens.)

Dr. Hauschka Skin Care: www.drhauschka.com
Jane Iredale mineral makeup: www.janeiredale.com

Supplements

All Clear Medicine products, including those for detoxification, general
health and hormonal benefits: www.shop.drnatashaturner.com
Dream Protein (all-natural whey protein supplement):
www.shop.drnatashaturner.com

Specialty Foods

Green & Blacks' organic chocolate: www.greenandblacks.com
NewTree fine Belgian dark chocolate: www.newtree.com
Camino organic fair-trade chocolate: www.lasiembra.com/camino
POM Wonderful pomegranate juice: www.pomwonderful.com
La Tortilla Factory pita, wraps and gluten-free products:
www.latortillafactory.com
Muzi Tea green tea: www.muzitea.com
Pita Gourmet Low Carb, High Protein Pita: www.eatpitagourmet.com
Organic Meadow organic pressed cottage cheese:
www.organicmeadow.com
Liberté organic yogurt (this brand has the right balance of protein and
carbs): http://liberte.ca
Dimpflmeier Bakery 100% rye bread: www.dimpflmeierbakery.com
Food for Life Baking Company Ezekiel breads: www.foodforlife.com
Bob's Red Mill gluten-free and other grain products: www.bobsredmill.
com
GP8 Oxygen Water: www.gp8.com

Relaxation Aids

HeartMath: www.heartmath.com

Toxin-Free Household Cleaning Products

Nature Clean: www.naturecleanliving.com
Attitude: www.labonneattitude.com
Seventh Generation: www.seventhgeneration.com

Water Filtration System

Nimbus Water Systems: www.nimbuswatersystems.com

Organic Cotton Bedding and Mattresses

Guide to Less Toxic Products (provides numerous sources):
www.lesstoxicguide.ca

Essentia Natural Memory Foam Mattresses: www.myessentia.com

Health Information Resources

Life Extension Foundation: www.lifeextensionfoundation.org

SeaChoice healthy seafood choices: www.seachoice.org

Harvard T.H. Chan School of Public Health, The Nutrition Source: www.hsph.harvard.edu/nutritionsource

Whole Foods Market (tasty soup recipes!): www.wholefoodsmarket.com/recipes

Environmental Working Group information about cosmetics, seafood safety, etc.: www.ewg.org

CalorieKing nutrition information database: www.calorieking.com

ACKNOWLEDGMENTS

Besides my first book, *The Hormone Diet*, this is my favorite. It has evolved to become my simplest, most effective plan yet. As always, a project of this nature is not possible without the help and support of many.

Thank you to my husband, Tim, for dealing with my time pressures and stress ☺. To my family—thank you for your support and encouragement.

Thank you to Brandy Ryan and to Linda Pruessen for your editing skills and thoughtful ideas. You both make me sound better, making my message to the reader approachable and clear.

Thank you to my agent, Rick Broadhead, for getting *The Hormone Boost* to publishers, for your fantastic attention to detail and your exemplary work ethic. Thank you to Pamela Murray and Anne Collins at Random House Canada and Jennifer Levesque at Rodale for your input and expertise (and for graciously agreeing to give an extension when I needed it!).

Thank you to my publicists Kaitlin Smith at Penguin Random House Canada and Emily Eagan at Rodale.

I would also like to offer gratitude to Suzanne Somers and Dr. Mehmet Oz for endorsing my work and for your continual efforts to bring preventative medicine to the forefront.

Thank you to Anthony Boudreau for your creation of the three Hormone Boost workout routines and to Jacqueline Ferretti for your input on the recipes. A huge thank-you to the rest of the team of staff and associates at Clear Medicine. Every day you inspire and guide people to live healthier, balanced lives. Your work is truly making a difference as you inspire the expansion of our philosophy for true wellness care.

Thank you to my patients and to the clients of Clear Medicine. It's my experience with you that keeps the Hormone Diet approach evolving.

And thank *you*, the reader, for picking up this book and for sharing your success stories. You have not only made a difference in your own life, but generously taken the time to provide the proof and necessary encouragement to so many others that change is possible—and doable! Thank you for helping me to achieve my goal of inspiring others to take responsibility for their health and to live healthier lives.

GENERAL INDEX

Note: Page numbers in italics indicate material in separate text boxes. Recipes are listed in the index following.

A

acetylcholine, 14, 72–76
  supplement options, 75–76
acetylcholinesterase, 203
acetyl-L-carnitine, 71, 75
ACTH (adrenocorticotropic
    hormone), 43
ADHD (attention deficit
    hyperactivity disorder), 115
adiponectin, 13, 79–88
  benefits, 80–88
  boosting, 88–90, 223
  and inflammation, 13, 79–80,
    81, 193, 205
  supplement options, 90–91
adrenal glands, 27, 33, 42–43. See
    also adrenalin; DHEA
adrenalin, 13, 42–49
  benefits, 43–46
  boosting, 46–47
  supplement options, 47–49
agave, 189
age, 11–12, 29, 82
ALA (alpha-linolenic acid), 203, 232
alarm clocks, 149, 151
alcohol, 172, 195. See also wine

alkalinization, 209
aluminum, 139
Alzheimer's disease, 67, 73, 203
amino acids, 101, 102. See also
    specific amino acids
  in diet, 186, 195
  as supplements, 70–71, 209–10
andropause, 57
angelica, 173–74
Anna A., 205–6
anthocyanins, 201
antibiotics, 10
antioxidants, 146, 201, 213–14
anxiety, 115
appetite, 103, 221
  factors affecting, 109–10, 147
  serotonin and, 111–13, 117
arginine, 63, 70
aromatherapy, 74
ashwagandha, 38–39, 155
athletes, 67–68, 71. See also
    exercise; workouts
autism spectrum disorder, 115
autonomic nervous system, 45–46
avocado oil, 83–84
avocados, 142

B

bacteria (gut), 32, 160
beauty products, 144–47
bedroom. *See also* sleep
　decluttering, 134–35, 150
　preparing, 147–56
beds and bedding, 150, 152
berries, 89, 193, 200–201
beta adrenergic receptors,
　24–25
beverages, 253. *See also specific*
　beverages
bipolar disorder, 115
bisphosphonates, 228
black cohosh, 173
blenders, 139–40
blood pressure, 201
blood sugar, 204, 225
　carbohydrates and, 93, 95
　hormones and, 13, 44, 102
blueberries, 89, 193, 200–201
BMR (basal metabolic rate), 24
bone health, 176, 226–33. *See also*
　osteoporosis
　density loss, 226–28, 230
　hormones and, 51–52, 122–23
　maintaining, 228–31
　supplement options, 231–33
Boudreau, Anthony, 226, 237
bowel function, 161–63
BPA (bisphenol A), 138
breakfast, 123–24, 187–88, 195,
　196, 204, 268
breast health, 176
butyrate, 202

C

caffeine, 172. *See also* coffee; tea
calcium-D-glucarate, 166
calories, 199, 219–20
cAMP, 39
cancer, 80

carbohydrates, 198. *See also* sugars;
　specific sources
　and blood sugar, 93, 95
　food choices, 248–50, 254–57
　high-glycemic, 96
　and hormone levels, 62, 112–13,
　　116–17
　and insulin levels, 93, 95
　low-glycemic, 97, 98, 186
　sensitivity to, 81, 98
　sources, 95–96, 99–100
　starchy, 117, 249–50, 255–56
　when to eat, 86, 89, 112–13, 187,
　　189
cardio training, 224, 234, 235
L-carnitine, 71, 75
carrots, 97
cereals, 99
chasteberry (vitex), 125, 175
cheese, 192, 202
chemical exposure, 61, 145, 152,
　171–72
chokeberries, 201
cholecystokinin (CCK), 112
cholesterol, 121, 176
　thyroid hormones and, 25, 28, 34
choline, 75–76
Chopra, Deepak, 53–54
1,8-cineole, 74
circadian clock, 119–21
circuit training, 233
Citrus aurantium, 48
CLA (conjugated linoleic acid), 83,
　204–5, 232, 235
cleaning products, 139
clutter. *See* decluttering
coconut oil, 142
coffee, 85, 89
coffee bean extract, 90
cognitive function
　food boosters, 200, 201, 203
　hormones and, 29–30, 31–32,
　　66–67, 114–15

Coleus forskohlii, 39
Commiphora mukul, 39
condiments, 252
conjugation, 165–66. See also
    detoxification
constipation, 32, 163
cookware, 139
cortisol, 33, 43, 46, 62. See also
    fight-or-flight response;
    stress
  hormones and, 27, 54, 116
creatine monohydrate, 235
curcumin (turmeric), 36, 85–86,
    90
currants (black), 201
cytokines, 85

D
dairy products, 101, 192
decluttering, 15–16, 134–36
Demeter, Mike, 225
depression, 31, 46, 57–58, 115. See
    also mood
detoxification, 164–66, 172,
    179–80, 216
DHA (docosahexaenoic acid), 115
DHEA (dehydroepiandrosterone),
    14, 50–56, 220
  benefits, 51–53, 63
  boosting, 53–54
  supplement options, 54–56,
    232–33
diabetes, 79–80, 84, 103–4. See
    also blood sugar; insulin
diarrhea, 32
diets, 84, 87. See also foods; meals;
    nutrition
  elimination, 179–80
  low-carbohydrate, 35, 62, 81
  Mediterranean, 228
  no-carbohydrate, 93–94
  starchy carb–free, 117

Supercharged Hormone, 34
  vegan/vegetarian, 261
digestion, 32–34, 159–63
dioxins, 138
DMAE (dimethylaminoethanol),
    76
dopamine, 15, 107–11, 117–18
  boosting, 123–24
  supplement options, 124–25
dysbiosis, 32

E
eczema, 179, 180
elderberries, 201
electromagnetic fields (EMFs), 149
Elizabeth R., 182
Emily B., 128–29
emollients, 146
Environmental Defence, 145
Environmental Working Group,
    144
EPA (eicosapentaenoic acid), 115
epinephrine. See adrenalin
estrogen, 67, 165–66, 170, 230
  preventing buildup, 63, 162, 220
exercise, 175, 194. See also
    workouts; specific types of
    exercise
  and acetylcholine, 72–73, 75
  and adiponectin, 84, 89
  and adrenalin, 44–45, 46, 47
  benefits, 219–21
  and DHEA, 54
  and dopamine, 124
  eating and, 195, 234
  and glucagon, 104
  and growth hormone, 67–68,
    69
  and mood, 220, 221
  scheduling, 135–36, 224
  and serotonin, 126
  supplement options, 235

exercise *(cont.)*
  and testosterone, 61, 62
  and thyroid hormones, 35–36, 37
  tracking, 317–18

F

fasting (intermittent), 89–90, 104
  benefits, 69–70, 82, 87–88
  supports for, 189–90, 215–16
fat (body), 102, 113–14, 122, 201,
    221
  adiponectin and, 81, 82
fatigue, 136
fat-loss six, 12–14, 23–105. *See also*
    specific hormones
  boosting, 216–17
fats (dietary), 198–99, 251, 258,
    262
  healthy, 82–84, 89, 186, 192, 215
  unhealthy, 191, 192
fertility, 53
fiber, 84, 88, 186, 262
  food sources, 198–99, 251–52,
    258
  supplement options, 162, 214–15
fight-or-flight response, 42–43. *See*
    also cortisol; stress
fish, 88, 190, 192
fish oil, 82, 230
flame retardants, 152
flour, 192
food processors, 140
foods. *See also* diets; meals;
    nutrition
  allergies to, 33, 178, 179–80
  to avoid, 137, 190–91, 192, 207
  containers for, 137–38, 142
  hormone-boosting, 192–93
  intolerances of, 33, 178–79
  permitted, 186–93, 200–205,
    245–64
  preparing, 138, 139, 141, 143–44

  shopping for, 143, 197–99,
    265–66
  tracking intake, 313–16
forskohlin, 39
Franco S., 105
fruit, 100, 192. *See also* berries;
    specific fruits
  choosing, 143, 193, 245, 256–57,
    260–61

G

GABA (gamma-aminobutyric
    acid), 156
GALT (gut-associated lymphoid
    tissue), 33
gastrin, 32–33
gastrointestinal system, 32–34,
    103, 159–63
  bacteria in, 32, 160
  bowel function, 161–63
German Body Composition
    Training (GBCT), 225–26
ghrelin, 147
GLP-1 (glucagon-like peptide-1),
    103, 204
glucagon, 13, 93–105
  benefits, 102–4
  boosting, 104
gluconeogenesis, 102
glucuronidation, 166. *See also*
    detoxification
glutamine, 70
glutathione, 166
glycemic index (GI), 96–98,
    99–100
glycemic load (GL), 97
L-alpha-glycerylphosphorylcholine
    (alpha-GPC), 71, 76
glycine, 71
glycogen, 44–45
glycogenolysis, 102
goiter, 36

greens, 200, 248–49, 254, 260
growth hormone, 14, 65–68, 77,
    116, 225
    benefits, 66–68
    boosting, 69–70
    supplement options, 70–72
gugulipids, 39
gut. *See* gastrointestinal system

H

hand sanitizer, 10
HCl (stomach acid), 33
heart disease, 28, 34–35, 203–4
hemp hearts, 192
herbs, 143, 259, 263
    phytoestrogenic, 173–74
    as supplements, 210–11
high-fructose corn syrup (HFCS),
    189
hippocampus, 57, 67
homocysteine, 34–35, 231
Hormone Boost, 5–6, 16–19. *See
    also* meals
    nutrition plan, 185–205
    preparing bathroom for,
        144–47
    preparing bedroom for, 147–56
    preparing body for, 159–81
    preparing home for, 133–58
    preparing kitchen for, 137–44
    success tracker, 313–19
    supplement plan, 212–17
    workout plan, 35–36, 85,
        219–42
hormones, 14–15, 220. See also
    specific hormones
    androgenic, 14, 50–64
    balancing, 93–94, 97
    and weight loss, 35–36, 44,
        58–59, 88, 108
5-HTP (5-hydroxytryptophan),
    126–27, 156, 230

hyperthyroidism (overactive
    thyroid), 32
hypogonadism, 57
hypothalamus, 43, 108, 112
hypothyroidism (underactive
    thyroid), 38

I

IgE antibodies, 178
IGF-1 (insulin-like growth factor 1),
    66, 71–72, 229–30
IgG antibodies/food allergies, 33,
    178–79, 180
immune system, 10, 45–46, 160,
    201
indole-3-carbinol (I3C), 165
inflammation, 115
    adiponectin and, 13, 79–80, 81,
        193, 205
    exercise and, 221, 222, 224
    of skin, 177, 179, 180
inositol, 127
insulin, 36, 84, 94, 231
    carbohydrates and, 93, 95
    protein and, 100, 101, 102
insulin index, 99–102
insulin resistance, 80–81, 84, 85.
    See also metabolic
    syndrome
iodine, 27, 38
iron supplements, 211
isoleucine, 101

J

Joanna B., 92

K

kitchen
    clearing out, 135, 137–44
    equipment for, 139–41
    pantry staples, 142
KonMari Method, 15–16

L

laughter, 70, 169–70
laundry products, 139
LDL (low-density lipoprotein), 25, 91. *See also* cholesterol
lecithin, 75–76
lemons, 142
leptin, 80, 85, 112, 147
leucine, 101
LH (luteinizing hormone), 63
licorice, 174
lifestyle, 175–76, 207
light, 119–21, 128, 148–49, 151
    natural, 61, 126, 154
limes, 142
Linda V., 77–78
linolenic acid, 83. *See also* ALA
liver, 102, 163–67, 169
longevity. *See* age
lubricants, 175–76
lycopene, 87
lysine, 71

M

macadamia nut oil, 83–84
magnesium glycinate, 155, 162–63, 173, 212–13
MariaLisa D., 64
Marilyn K., 49
Marlene W., 19–20
Mason jars, 140
massage, 124, 126, 169
Matheson, Jeff, 173
mattresses, 152
meals, 144, 199
    cheat, 191–92
    daily schedule for, 196–97
    grab-and-go, 267–69
    Meal 1, 123–24, 187–88, 195, 196, 204, 268
    Meal 2, 196–97, 268–69
    Meal 4, 197

on-the-go, 269–73
replacements for, 214–15, 263–64
timing, 112–13, 188, 194–95
meat, 141, 143, 190
meditation, 53–54, 126, 167–69
melatonin, 15, 115–23. *See also* tryptophan
    boosting, 127–28
    light and, 119–21, 128, 148–49, 151
    as supplement, 128, 156, 175, 232
memory, 8–9, 66–67
menopause, 31–32, 171, 172, 220. *See also* andropause
    supplement options, 173–75
Mercola, Joseph, 141
mercury contamination, 192
metabolic syndrome, 203. *See also* insulin resistance
metabolism, 9, 35–36
    thyroid hormones and, 24–25, 28
methylation, 165–66. *See also* detoxification
Michelle C., 217–18
microwaves, 138, 141
mindfulness, 144. *See also* meditation
minerals, 146, 209–10, 211, 232
mitochondria, 84
mood, 10–11, 136. *See also* depression
    boosters, 106–29, 200, 220, 221
    hormones and, 29–30, 31, 46, 57–58
muscles, 194, 220
    hormones and, 44–45, 52–53, 60–61, 67–68, 84
music, 47, 235

N

neuropeptides, 112, 177
neurotransmitters, 107. *See also* acetylcholine; dopamine; melatonin; serotonin

nightclothes, 153
noradrenalin (NA), 43
nutrition, 172, 207–8. *See also*
diets; food; meals
and acetylcholine, 75
and adiponectin, 88, 89
for adrenalin boost, 46
for dopamine boost, 123–24
and glucagon, 104
and growth hormone, 69
for melatonin boost, 127
for serotonin boost, 125
and skin health, 179–80
for thyroid health, 37–38
nuts, 192, 203

O

obesity, 103, 110. *See also* weight
gain; weight loss
oils (in diet), 83, 142, 191, 204–5.
See also specific oils
choosing, 251, 258, 265
olive oil, 83, 142, 192, 205, 215
omega-3 fatty acids, 88, 114–15
as supplements, 173, 181, 213, 232
organization, 15–16, 134–36
orgasms. *See* sex
ornithine, 70
osteocalcin, 230–31
osteopenia, 226
osteoporosis, 52, 122, 226–28. *See
also* bone health
overeating, 135

P

Parkinson's disease, 107
PCOS (polycystic ovary syndrome),
51
peanuts, 191
pears, 192, 201–2
phenols, 202
phenylalanine, 125

phosphatidylcholine (lecithin),
75–76
pH testing, 209
phthalates, 137–38
phytochemicals, 87
phytoestrogens, 172, 173–74
Pick-4 salads, 254–59
Pick-4 smoothies, 260–64
pineal gland, 148, 149. *See also*
melatonin
pituitary gland, 27, 43
plastics, 137–38
PMS (premenstrual syndrome),
125, 175
Poliquin, Charles, 113, 225
polyphenols, 202, 203–4
PPARs (peroxisome proliferator-
activated receptors), 221
pregnancy, 30–31, 76, 202
probiotics, 160, 162, 173, 181, 213
progesterone, 125, 175, 230
protein, 198
and hormone levels, 62, 94–95,
112, 116, 127
insulin effects, 100, 101, 102
intake guidelines, 186–87,
261–62
sources, 192, 246–48, 257–58
supplemental, 104, 214, 247–48
vegetarian sources, 264
when to eat, 195
from whey, 188, 192, 204
protein bars, 215, 247–48, 263
psoriasis, 180
pterostilbene, 201

Q

quercetin, *58*

R

Rambie, Hala, 225
red clover, 174

Relora, 55, 154–55, 232–33
resistance training, *194*, 220
resistin, 80–81, 85
resveratrol, 86, 91
rhodiola, 125, 127
Rivers, Mary, 226
rosemary oil, 74, 76
royal jelly, 56
rT3 (reverse triiodothyronine), 26, 27

S

safflower oil, 83, 204–5
sage/sage oil, 73, 76, 174
St. John's wort, 127
salads, 254–59
salmon, 189
salt, 142, 198–99
sarcopenia, 52–53
sauces, 143
schizophrenia, 115
sclerostin, 229–30
screen time, 121
seasonal affective disorder (SAD), 116–17
selenium, 27, 38, 39
serotonin, 15, 31, 111–15
    boosting, 125–26, 230
    carbohydrates and, 112–13, 116–17
    peripheral, 114, 159
    supplement options, 126–27
    tryptophan and, 111, 112, 115
sex, 54, 61, 124, 149–50, 170–76
Sharon and Ross, 157–58
Sharon S., 40–41
skin, 176–81. *See also* skin care
    inflammation of, 177, 179, 180
    supplement options, 181
skin care, 144–47, 178
    natural products for, 146–47, 179, 181

sleep, 147, 153–54. *See also* bedroom
    acetylcholine and, 73–75
    and hormones, 37, 54, 61, 69
    light and, 119–21, 148–49, 151, 153
    melatonin and, 118–19, 127
    supplement options, 154–56
slow cookers, 140
smoking, 175
smoothies, 214–15, 260–64
snacks, 100, 188–89, 197, 268–69
sodium. *See* salt
soups, 143
soy, 87
spices, 142, 252, 259, 263
spiralizers, 141
sports, 62. *See also* exercise
SSRIs (selective serotonin reuptake inhibitors), 31, 230
stevia, 189
stomach acid (HCl), 33
stool testing, *161*
strength, 8, 60–61. *See also* muscles
strength training, *68*, 224–26. *See also* weight training
    benefits, 224, 229–30
    frequency, 89, 233–34
    workouts, 237–41
stress. *See also* cortisol; fight-or-flight response
    clutter and, 136
    effects, 45, 112, 177–78
    exercise and, 220, 222
    hormones and, 54, 67, 69
    managing, 167–70, 176, 180, 318
    and thyroid function, 33, 37
sugars, 95–96, 190, 192. *See also* carbohydrates
sulfation, 166. *See also* detoxification
sunlight, 61, 126, 154

sunscreens, 145
The Supercharged Hormone Diet
(Turner), 163
superfoods, 200–205
supplements, 207–17, *See also*
specific hormones
foundation products, 212–16
herbal, 210–11
intake guidelines, 211
optimizing, 208–11
sweeteners (artificial), 189
synephrine, 48

T

T3 (triiodothyronine), 12–13, 25–26,
35–36. *See also* rT3
as mood booster, 29–30, 31
T4 (thyroxine), 12–13, 25, 29–30,
32
tea, 203–4
green, 85, 91, 203
herbal, 189, 215–16
television, 121, 149
temperature, 126, 150–51
testosterone, 14, 56–63
benefits, 52–53, 57–61, 171, 230
boosting, 61–62
deficiency of, 56, 171–72
sex and, 61, 170
supplement options, 62–63
thyroid gland, 27, 28–30. *See also*
thyroid hormones
thyroid hormones, 12–13, 23–41.
See also T3; T4; TSH
benefits, 31–36
boosting, 37–38
and cholesterol, 25, 28, 34
and metabolism, 24–25, 28
pregnancy and, 30–31
supplement options, 30, 38–40
tests for, 29, 30
toaster ovens, 141
tomatoes, 87, 89

tomato juice, 192–93
trans fatty acids, 191
transit-time test, *161*
Tribulus terrestris (puncture vine),
63
tryptophan, 116, 125, 127
and serotonin, 111, 112, 115
TSH (thyroid-stimulating
hormone), 12–13, 25, 32
turmeric (curcumin), 36, 85–86,
90
Turner, Natasha, 1–5, 30
"TurnTash Method", 15–16, 134
L-tyrosine, 27, 38, 39
as supplement, 48–49, 71,
124–25

V

vaginal dryness, 175–76
valine, 101
vegetables, 200, 248–49, 254, 260
vinegars, 142
vitamins, 208, 209–11, 232
B vitamins, 34–35, 47, 111, 127,
231
vitamin C, 48, 163, 166, 181, 232
vitamin D, 114–15, 208, 230, 231
vitamin E, 173, 181, 214, 232
vitamin K, 200, 211
vitex (chasteberry), 125, 175

W

walking, 89, 223, 234, 237
walnuts, 203
water (drinking), 138, 167, 193
weight gain, 28, 112, 121–22, 160,
191
weight loss, 48
hormones and, 35–36, 44,
58–59, 88, 108
sleep and, 147–48
tracking, 314–15, 317

weight training, 54, 225, 235–36, 237. *See also* strength training
whey protein, 188, 192, 204
white noise, 151
wine (red), 58, 86, 117
workouts, 233–35, 236. *See also* exercise
  equipment, 234–35
  terms used, 238–39

weekly schedule, 221–22, 236–37, 239–41

Y

yoga, 85, 89, 222–23, 234, 237
yogurt, 142

Z

zinc, 63, 90–91, 212

RECIPE INDEX

A

almond milk. *See also different flavors (below)*
  Apple Pie Smoothie, 306
  Blueberry Spinach Smoothie, Dr. Turner's Favorite, 310
  Café au Lait, 310
  Carrot Cake Smoothie, 312
  Choco Banana-rama Smoothie, 305
  Matcha Madness Smoothie, 306
  Pear and Basil Smoothie, 308
almond milk, chocolate
  Cocoa Hemp Cinna-Bliss Smoothie, 307
  Dark Chocolate Salty Crunch Smoothie, 311
almond milk, vanilla
  Banana "Cream Pie" Smoothie, 307
  Gingerbread Smoothie, 308
  Greena-Colada, 311
  Mint Chocolate Chip Smoothie, 310
  Pumpkin Pie Smoothie, 307
  Snickerdoodle Cashew Smoothie, 311
  Strawberry Ginger Turmarika Smoothie, 309

Apple Pie Smoothie, 306
Asian Sirloin Steak, 291
asparagus
  Baked Salmon and Asparagus in Foil, 274
  Flank Steak with Romesco Sauce and Cauliflower Mash, 293
avocado
  Chicken Fajita Lettuce Wraps, Sepherha's, 278
  Green Leap Avocado Smoothie, 309
  Healthy Cobb Salad, 283
  Mint Chocolate Chip Smoothie, 310
  Protein Pancakes, 269
  Quick and Easy Mason Jar Salad, 271
  Rainbow Thai Chicken Salad, 275
  Tuna Power Bowl, 286

B

bacon (turkey)
  Egg Pepper Pockets with Turkey Bacon, 285
  Healthy Cobb Salad, 283

bananas
    Banana "Cream Pie" Smoothie,
        307
    Choco Banana-rama Smoothie,
        305
    Gingerbread Smoothie, 308
    Protein Pancakes, 269
basil
    Betta Bruschetta Chicken, 287
    Pear and Basil Smoothie, 308
    Spicy Basil Zucchini Pasta with
        Pecan-Crusted Chicken,
        281
beans and lentils
    Chicken and Lentil Chard Soup,
        297
    Turmeric and Cannellini Bean
        Stew, 295
    Tuscan One-Pot Halibut, 298
beef
    Asian Sirloin Steak, 291
    Fake-Out Takeout Beef and
        Broccoli, 304
    Flank Steak with Romesco
        Sauce and Cauliflower
        Mash, 293
    Slow Cooker Beef Stew, 300
    Zucchini Pasta and Turkey Rosé
        Sauce, 292

C
cabbage
    Deconstructed Cod Taco Salad,
        282
    Lemon Tamari Chicken Salad,
        273
    Rainbow Thai Chicken Salad,
        275
cacao powder/nibs. See chocolate
    and cacao
Café au Lait, 310
carrots
    Carrot Cake Smoothie, 312

Chicken and Lentil Chard Soup,
    297
One-Pot Paprika Chicken, 301
Rainbow Thai Chicken Salad,
    275
Slow Cooker Beef Stew, 300
Thai Turkey Lettuce Wraps,
    272
Turmeric and Cannellini Bean
    Stew, 295
Zucchini Pasta and Turkey Rosé
    Sauce, 292
cashew milk. See almond milk
cauliflower
    Flank Steak with Romesco
        Sauce and Cauliflower
        Mash, 293
    Paella and Cauliflower Rice,
        294
    Pan-Seared Scallops with
        Cauliflower Mash and
        Spinach, 284
    Turmeric and Cannellini Bean
        Stew, 295
celery
    Coconut Curry Butternut
        Chicken Soup, 302
    Slow Cooker Beef Stew, 300
    Spinach Salad with Grilled
        Chicken, Sassy, 277
    Zucchini Pasta and Turkey Rosé
        Sauce, 292
cheese
    Cast-Iron Eggy Bake with
        Ricotta, 289
    Oven-Baked Goat Cheese,
        Tomato and Spinach
        Omelet, 289
    Stuffed Peppers, 296
chicken. See also turkey
    Betta Bruschetta Chicken, 287
    Chicken and Lentil Chard Soup,
        297

Chicken and Yogurt Curry,
Jackie's, 280
Chicken Fajita Lettuce Wraps,
Sepherha's, 278
Coconut Curry Butternut
Chicken Soup, 302
Healthy Cobb Salad, 283
Lemon Tamari Chicken Salad,
273
Mediterranean Chicken, Sunny,
276
Mushroom Chicken Quinoa
Risotto, 302
One-Pot Paprika Chicken, 301
Quick and Easy Mason Jar
Salad, 271
Rainbow Thai Chicken Salad,
275
Rosemary Chicken with Sautéed
Rapini, Comforting, 276
Spicy Basil Zucchini Pasta with
Pecan-Crusted Chicken,
281
Spinach Salad with Grilled
Chicken, Sassy, 277
Turmeric and Cannellini Bean
Stew, 295
chocolate and cacao
Café au Lait, 310
Choco Banana-rama Smoothie,
305
Chocolate Cherry Delight, 308
Cocoa Hemp Cinna-Bliss
Smoothie, 307
Dark Chocolate Salty Crunch
Smoothie, 311
Mint Chocolate Chip Smoothie,
310
cilantro
Chicken and Yogurt Curry,
Jackie's, 280
Chicken Fajita Lettuce Wraps,
Sepherha's, 278

Rainbow Thai Chicken Salad,
275
cinnamon
Blueberry Spinach Smoothie,
Dr. Turner's Favorite, 310
Carrot Cake Smoothie, 312
Cocoa Hemp Cinna-Bliss
Smoothie, 307
Snickerdoodle Cashew
Smoothie, 311
Cobb Salad, Healthy, 283
coconut
Carrot Cake Smoothie, 312
Greena-Colada, 311
coconut milk
Chocolate Cherry Delight,
308
Coconut Curry Butternut
Chicken Soup, 302
Green Leap Avocado Smoothie,
309
Peach-Colada Smoothie, 306
Snickerdoodle Cashew
Smoothie, 311
Zucchini Pasta and Turkey Rosé
Sauce, 292
Cod Taco Salad, Deconstructed,
282
cucumber
Lemon Tamari Chicken Salad,
273
Quick and Easy Mason Jar
Salad, 271
Sassy Spinach Salad with
Grilled Chicken, 277
Tuna Power Bowl, 286

D

Deconstructed Cod Taco Salad,
282
Dr. Turner's Favorite Blueberry
Spinach Smoothie, 310

E

eggs
  Cast-Iron Eggy Bake with
      Ricotta, 289
  Egg Pepper Pockets with Turkey
      Bacon, 285
  Oven-Baked Goat Cheese,
      Tomato and Spinach
      Omelet, 289
  Protein Pancakes, 269
  Spinach-Mushroom Crustless
      Quiche Cups, 270
  Zucchini Pancakes, 270

F

Fake-Out Takeout Beef and
    Broccoli, 304
fiber supplements. *See* smoothies
fish. *See also* seafood
  Baked Salmon and Asparagus in
      Foil, 274
  Deconstructed Cod Taco Salad,
      282
  Salmon Patties with Simple
      Tartar Sauce, 288
  Sole with Zucchini and Olives,
      Sassy, 290
  Tuna Power Bowl, 286
  Tuscan One-Pot Halibut, 298
Flank Steak with Romesco Sauce
    and Cauliflower Mash,
    293
fruit
  Apple Pie Smoothie, 306
  Blueberry Spinach Smoothie,
      Dr. Turner's Favorite, 310
  Chocolate Cherry Delight, 308
  Matcha Madness Smoothie, 306
  Peach-Colada Smoothie, 306
  Pear and Basil Smoothie, 308
  Strawberry Ginger Turmarika
      Smoothie, 309

G

garlic
  Asian Sirloin Steak, 291
  Betta Bruschetta Chicken, 287
  Chicken and Lentil Chard Soup,
      297
  Chicken and Yogurt Curry,
      Jackie's, 280
  Chicken Fajita Lettuce Wraps,
      Sepherha's, 278
  Flank Steak with Romesco
      Sauce and Cauliflower
      Mash, 293
  Mushroom Chicken Quinoa
      Risotto, 302
  Paella and Cauliflower Rice,
      294
  Rosemary Chicken with Sautéed
      Rapini, Comforting, 276
  Squash Nest Spicy Garlic
      Shrimp, 299
  Zucchini Pasta and Turkey Rosé
      Sauce, 292
ginger
  Asian Sirloin Steak, 291
  Chicken and Yogurt Curry,
      Jackie's, 280
  Gingerbread Smoothie, 308
greens. *See also* kale; lettuce;
    spinach
  Chicken and Lentil Chard Soup,
      297
  Egg Pepper Pockets with Turkey
      Bacon, 285
  Greena-Colada, 311
  Green Leap Avocado Smoothie,
      309
  Quick and Easy Mason Jar
      Salad, 271
  Rosemary Chicken with Sautéed
      Rapini, Comforting, 276
  Tuna Power Bowl, 286

H
Healthy Cobb Salad, 283
hemp seeds
  Banana "Cream Pie" Smoothie,
    307
  Blueberry Spinach Smoothie,
    Dr. Turner's Favorite, 310
  Café au Lait, 310
  Chocolate Cherry Delight, 308
  Cocoa Hemp Cinna-Bliss
    Smoothie, 307
  Gingerbread Smoothie, 308
  Greena-Colada, 311
  Green Leap Avocado Smoothie,
    309
  Matcha Madness Smoothie, 306
  Peach-Colada Smoothie, 306
  Pumpkin Pie Smoothie, 307
  Snickerdoodle Cashew
    Smoothie, 311
  Strawberry Ginger Turmarika
    Smoothie, 309

J
Jackie's Chicken and Yogurt Curry,
  280

K
kale. *See also* greens
  Chocolate Cherry Delight, 308
  Greena-Colada, 311
  Green Leap Avocado Smoothie,
    309
  Tuna Power Bowl, 286

L
Lemon Tamari Chicken Salad,
  273
lettuce. *See also* greens
  Chicken Fajita Lettuce Wraps,
    Sepherha's, 278

Healthy Cobb Salad, 283
Thai Turkey Lettuce Wraps,
  272

M
Mason Jar Salad, Quick and Easy,
  271
Matcha Madness Smoothie, 306
Meals 1, 2 and 3 (starchy carb–free)
  recipes, 272–95
Meal 4 (starchy carb) recipes,
  295–304
Mediterranean Chicken, Sunny,
  276
milk (nondairy). *See* almond milk;
  coconut milk
Mint Chocolate Chip Smoothie,
  310
mushrooms
  Mushroom Chicken Quinoa
    Risotto, 302
  One-Pot Paprika Chicken, 301
  Spinach-Mushroom Crustless
    Quiche Cups, 270
  Thai Turkey Lettuce Wraps, 272
  Tuscan One-Pot Halibut, 298

N
nut butters
  Apple Pie Smoothie, 306
  Café au Lait, 310
  Choco Banana-rama Smoothie,
    305
  Dark Chocolate Salty Crunch
    Smoothie, 311
  Snickerdoodle Cashew
    Smoothie, 311
nuts
  Carrot Cake Smoothie, 312
  Green Leap Avocado Smoothie,
    309

nuts *(cont.)*
    Pear and Basil Smoothie, 308
    Spicy Basil Zucchini Pasta with
        Pecan-Crusted Chicken,
        281

O

One-Pot Paprika Chicken, 301
on-the-go recipes, 269–73

P

Paella and Cauliflower Rice, 294
pancakes, 269–70
Peach-Colada Smoothie, 306
Pear and Basil Smoothie, 308
peppers
    Betta Bruschetta Chicken, 287
    Cast-Iron Eggy Bake with
        Ricotta, 289
    Chicken Fajita Lettuce Wraps,
        Sepherha's, 278
    Deconstructed Cod Taco Salad,
        282
    Egg Pepper Pockets with Turkey
        Bacon, 285
    Flank Steak with Romesco
        Sauce and Cauliflower
        Mash, 293
    Mediterranean Chicken, Sunny,
        276
    Paella and Cauliflower Rice, 294
    Quick and Easy Mason Jar
        Salad, 271
    Rainbow Thai Chicken Salad,
        275
    Stuffed Peppers, 296
    Turmeric and Cannellini Bean
        Stew, 295
Pick-4-Salads
    dressing ingredients, 259
    ingredient choices, 254–58
Pick-4-Smoothies, 260–64

potatoes
    One-Pot Paprika Chicken, 301
    Slow Cooker Beef Stew, 300
Protein Pancakes, 269
protein powder. *See* smoothies
Pumpkin Pie Smoothie, 307
pumpkin seeds
    Quick and Easy Mason Jar
        Salad, 271
    Sassy Spinach Salad with
        Grilled Chicken, 277

Q

Quiche Cups, Spinach-Mushroom
    Crustless, 270
Quick and Easy Mason Jar Salad,
    271
quinoa
    Mushroom Chicken Quinoa
        Risotto, 302
    One-Pot Paprika Chicken, 301
    Stuffed Peppers, 296
    Turmeric and Cannellini Bean
        Stew, 295
    Tuscan One-Pot Halibut, 298

R

Rainbow Thai Chicken Salad, 275

S

salads
    dressing ingredients, 259
    ingredient choices, 254–58
salmon
    Baked Salmon and Asparagus in
        Foil, 274
    Salmon Patties with Simple
        Tartar Sauce, 288
seafood. *See also* fish
    Paella and Cauliflower Rice,
        294
    Pan-Seared Scallops with

Cauliflower Mash and
Spinach, 284
Squash Nest Spicy Garlic
Shrimp, 299
Sepherha's Chicken Fajita Lettuce
Wraps, 278
Slow Cooker Beef Stew, 300
smoothies, 260–64, 304–12
Snickerdoodle Cashew Smoothie,
311
Sole with Zucchini and Olives,
Sassy, 290
soups, 297, 302
spinach. *See also* greens
Betta Bruschetta Chicken, 287
Blueberry Spinach Smoothie,
Dr. Turner's Favorite, 310
Greena-Colada, 311
Green Leap Avocado Smoothie,
309
Oven-Baked Goat Cheese,
Tomato and Spinach
Omelet, 289
Pan-Seared Scallops with
Cauliflower Mash and
Spinach, 284
Peach-Colada Smoothie, 306
Sassy Spinach Salad with
Grilled Chicken, 277
Spinach-Mushroom Crustless
Quiche Cups, 270
squash. *See also* zucchini
Coconut Curry Butternut
Chicken Soup, 302
Pumpkin Pie Smoothie, 307
Squash Nest Spicy Garlic
Shrimp, 299
starchy carb–free recipes, 269–95
starchy carb recipes, 295–304
strawberries
Matcha Madness Smoothie, 306
Strawberry Ginger Turmarika
Smoothie, 309

T

Thai Chicken Salad, Rainbow, 275
Thai Turkey Lettuce Wraps, 272
tomatoes. *See also* tomatoes,
cherry/grape
Betta Bruschetta Chicken, 287
Cast-Iron Eggy Bake with
Ricotta, 289
Chicken and Lentil Chard Soup,
297
Chicken and Yogurt Curry,
Jackie's, 280
Chicken Fajita Lettuce Wraps,
Sepherha's, 278
Healthy Cobb Salad, 283
Mediterranean Chicken, Sunny,
276
Paella and Cauliflower Rice,
294
Slow Cooker Beef Stew, 300
Spinach Salad with Grilled
Chicken, Sassy, 277
Squash Nest Spicy Garlic
Shrimp, 299
Turmeric and Cannellini Bean
Stew, 295
Zucchini Pasta and Turkey Rosé
Sauce, 292
tomatoes, cherry/grape
Flank Steak with Romesco
Sauce and Cauliflower
Mash, 293
Oven-Baked Goat Cheese,
Tomato and Spinach
Omelet, 289
Quick and Easy Mason Jar
Salad, 271
Sassy Sole with Zucchini and
Olives, 290
Tuna Power Bowl, 286
turkey. *See also* chicken
Stuffed Peppers, 296
Thai Turkey Lettuce Wraps, 272

Zucchini Pasta and Turkey Rosé
   Sauce, 292
turmeric
   Strawberry Ginger Turmarika
      Smoothie, 309
   Turmeric and Cannellini Bean
      Stew, 295
Tuscan One-Pot Halibut, 298

V

vegetables. See also greens;
   specific vegetables
   Fake-Out Takeout Beef and
      Broccoli, 304
   Healthy Cobb Salad, 283
   Lemon Tamari Chicken Salad,
      273

Y

yogurt (Greek)
   Chicken and Yogurt Curry,
      Jackie's, 280
   Chicken Fajita Lettuce Wraps,
      Sepherha's, 278
   Coconut Curry Butternut
      Chicken Soup, 302

Deconstructed Cod Taco Salad,
   282
Healthy Cobb Salad, 283
Pumpkin Pie Smoothie, 307
Squash Nest Spicy Garlic
   Shrimp, 299
Zucchini Pancakes, 270

Z

zucchini
   Chicken Fajita Lettuce Wraps,
      Sepherha's, 278
   Mediterranean Chicken, Sunny,
      276
   Rosemary Chicken with Sautéed
      Rapini, Comforting,
      276
   Sassy Sole with Zucchini and
      Olives, 290
   Spicy Basil Zucchini Pasta with
      Pecan-Crusted Chicken,
      281
   Stuffed Peppers, 296
   Zucchini Pancakes, 270
   Zucchini Pasta and Turkey Rosé
      Sauce, 292

DR. NATASHA TURNER is a *New York Times* bestselling author and one of North America's leading naturopathic doctors, a sought-after speaker, a natural health expert and the founder of Clear Medicine Wellness Boutique in Toronto. In 2014 she was recognized by her professional organization as a leader in her field and in 2016 was awarded the top spot on a list of North America's Most Innovative Health Experts. Dr. Turner has been referred to as a friend of the *Dr. Oz Show* by Dr. Oz and is also a regular guest on the *Marilyn Denis Show*.